P9-DVV-117

Everything Left
to Remember

Also by Steph Jagger

Unbound: A Story of Snow and Self-Discovery

Everything Left to Remember

My Mother, Our Memories,
and a Journey Through the Rocky Mountains

Steph Jagger

FLATIRON
BOOKS
NEW YORK

EVERYTHING LEFT TO REMEMBER. Copyright © 2022 by Stephanie
Jagger. All rights reserved. Printed in the United States of
America. For information, address Flatiron Books,
120 Broadway, New York, NY 10271.

www.flatironbooks.com

Designed by Donna Sinisgalli Noetzel

Library of Congress Cataloging-in-Publication Data

Names: Jagger, Steph, author.
Title: Everything left to remember : my mother, our memories, and
  a journey through the Rocky Mountains / Steph Jagger.
Other titles: My mother, our memories, and a journey through the
  Rocky Mountains
Description: First edition. | New York, NY : Flatiron Books, 2022. |
Identifiers: LCCN 2021041626 | ISBN 9781250261830 (hardcover) |
  ISBN 9781250261854 (ebook)
Subjects: LCSH: Jagger, Steph—Family. | Alzheimer's disease—
  Patients—Care. | Alzheimer's disease—Patients—Family
  relationships—British Columbia—Vancouver. | Mothers and
  daughters—British Columbia—Vancouver. | Jagger, Steph—
  Travel—Montana. | Yellowstone National Park. | Glacier
  National Park (Mont.) | Grand Teton National Park (Wyo.) |
  Vancouver (B.C.)—Biography.
Classification: LCC RC523.2 .J335 2022 | DDC 362.1968/311—dc23
LC record available at https://lccn.loc.gov/2021041626

Our books may be purchased in bulk for promotional,
educational, or business use. Please contact your local
bookseller or the Macmillan Corporate and Premium Sales
Department at 1-800-221-7945, extension 5442, or by email at
MacmillanSpecialMarkets@macmillan.com.

First Edition: 2022

10 9 8 7 6 5 4 3 2 1

For my mother.

The way you revealed yourself in the midst of your disappearance has taught me more than the sun, and the moon, and the swing of the ocean between them.

Good God, how you've set us all free.

Contents

We have instructions and a map buried in our hearts when we enter this world.

—JOY HARJO

Everything Left
to Remember

Introduction

Picking Up Leaves

My mother has a story, one she's been carrying with her since 1966, a tale she tucked firmly inside of herself. She also has Alzheimer's. And from the moment she was diagnosed, I sensed those two things—the disease and the story—were somehow inextricable. They seemed woven together into a thick cord, and I felt if I could only untangle them, it might help set her free.

I came into this world with my mother's story written into the supercoil of my DNA. Like a dormant seed placed in deep soil, transferred somehow from her garden to mine. Every word of it was imprinted onto my biopolymer strands. I'm certain of it. It ran through my blood before it was blood. It was drilled into my marrow before I had bones.

It was part of my contract, the fine print that the Universe, and my mother, and little bits of my soul haggled over before agreeing to drop me into her arms.

My mother would never utter much more than a word or two about it—the child she conceived with my father well before they were married, the subsequent adoption that took place, and the decades-long cover-up of their teenage faux pas. Nor would she discuss the emotions involved—if, when, or how they had ever arrived. Her lifelong dislike of words would never have let her; nor, eventually, would Alzheimer's. So they gave the story to me. It was part of my inheritance.

Growing up, I didn't know the telling of her story would be my job. I wasn't walking around as a twelve-year-old thinking this was my raison d'être—I figured that was more along the lines of "wear jelly shoes and tell people what to do." (Somewhere along the way, I developed a healthy dose of self-assurance and an audacious kind of bravery, but that's beside the point.)

The realization arrived about twenty-five years later when I was walking through the woods with my mother, when she paused on the trail and told me exactly what I was to do.

It was a clear day in early November, streams of misty light were moving through the forest, and big-leaf maples were dropping red-and-yellow clues about where we were and where we might go next.

"What do you think about me writing a book about us?" I asked, as we turned onto my favorite section of trail. "About you?"

"A book about me?!" she said in surprise. "But there's nothing terribly interesting about me."

And then she paused, mid-stride. She was thinking about something. As of late, watching her do this was not unlike watching a small child with an Imbucare Box, a slow and imprecise process of trying to fit the blue block into the hole made for the blue block, before moving on to the small red square.

"Would I . . ." she said, the question forming slowly in her brain. "Would I have to write any of it?"

"No, Mom," I said. "You don't have to write a single word."

She looked over to me and I saw the small muscles in her face relax. She smiled at me, reached out, and took both of my hands in hers.

"Oh, good," she said, while squeezing them. "I'll walk it. You write it."

And with that she stepped forward, resuming her stride.

I thought for sure she would say more, but she didn't.

We wound our way through a grove of especially large maples, a scattering of their leaves laying here and there on the ground. I picked one up and handed it to my mom like it was a big orange balloon on a string. It didn't take long for her to start in on a game of peekaboo, using the leaf to cover her face before quickly peeking forward with a cuckoo type of sound.

"Here I am!" she said with a laugh.

When she did it a second time the leaf fell out of her hand and fluttered to the ground. I bent over, picked it up off the trail, and handed it back to her.

"That's what you were made for," she said, an unusual lucidity in her voice.

"For what?" I asked.

"For picking up all the leaves I've dropped."

Shortly after my mother's diagnosis, and well prior to this walk in the woods, my mother and I had taken a trip together—two weeks on the road, driving through and camping in a handful of national parks. At the time, I had a desperate sense of urgency to know more about her life, to know all of my mother. The idea of Alzheimer's taking pieces of her away before I had the whole picture was unbearable to me. Especially because I'd always sensed that some pieces of her had long been missing.

There was so much I didn't understand about my mother. There was a specific section of the puzzle from 1966 that felt very unknown to me—what had happened leading up to, and after, the birth of my eldest brother. But there was also what felt like a general veil of withholding.

I didn't have a name for this. I didn't have words for what I felt was being held back. But I had a sensation, and over the years it had told me, time and time again, that some part of my mother was, and had always been, inaccessible to me, perhaps even to her.

The ache to know more of my mother had existed within me for a long time, but something about it changed when she was diagnosed—a dull and muted pain was replaced with something more searing.

I wanted to know all of her—who she'd been, what she'd felt, the sum of all her parts—and this trip together felt like my last chance, a brief moment in time where my mother had lost a bit of her filter, but still retained the shape of her mind.

So I reached for her hand, and together, we walked into the wilderness.

Sometimes we're given the stories of our mothers and fathers, of our ancestors before them, and the ones who came before that. Bundles of words, written or spoken aloud, that tell us where we come from and who they really were, what kind of sand and silt they were made of. Other times we have to let the stories rise up from the soil within and around us, from the places they were buried, laid to rest. We have to watch for them as they float through the air—the tiny spores of them dispersed into the atmosphere after the storms come rolling through, covering us in a fine mist, in something we can barely detect.

I didn't know how to translate a story that didn't have words. I didn't know how to pick up those leaves, how to parse them out, to differentiate between them and the air I was breathing. But she gave me the answers. For the key to unlocking it all was the language, the fluency of wordlessness she taught me on our journey together, everything that lives inside of a hush.

The deal was clear. My mother was to live it, I was to write it.

It would be an instruction manual, a guide of sorts for my mother's freedom. What I didn't know at the time was that it also held instructions for my own.

1

A Family Constellation

It took me eleven months to notice the tear in the fabric, and seven words for it to rip straight down the middle. Eleven months and seven words.

In June of 2015, my mother was diagnosed with Alzheimer's. This was what first snagged the fabric of us—the nail that caught, and then pulled on, the veins and small threads that made up the garment.

At the time, I had very little understanding of how deeply my mother and I had been woven together, of how intricately her seams had been stitched into mine, or how the pulling on one would lead to the unraveling of another.

I told myself I could handle her falling apart at the seams

and synapses. I told myself that my seams and synapses would not be affected. I did so with the kind of confidence that comes from not knowing much about anything.

It would take me eleven months to realize this was not true. To see that the flood of questions I had about my mother's dying were directly linked to the questions I had about my own living. To see the layers of anger that lived, unnamed and unexpressed, between those two places.

It would take me until the moment my therapist, Sara, said the most obvious and painful thing to me: "You think you're bigger than your mother."

I heard the fabric as it ripped. I immediately looked away from Sara. I felt my eyes pin themselves to my shoes. It's a rather difficult thing, you know, to make eye contact as you feel yourself come apart.

I don't know how many seconds or minutes passed by, but at some point she said it again: "You think you're bigger than your mother."

There was no question for me to answer, but I knew she was waiting for confirmation, for some sign that I knew what she'd said was true.

My body began to move, to answer for itself, well before my brain had a chance to make sense of what Sara had said. Tears slid out of my downcast eyes. My insides shifted, as waves rolled from one side of my stomach to the other. The only thing that kept me standing was the tension in my shoulders, pulling upward, and upward again.

I bit the inside edge of my lower lip as my body brimmed

with discomfort. Sara's eyes caught mine, and as they did, I felt another tear slide down my face.

"Thought so," she said.

I gently rocked on my feet. It was a subtle heel-to-toe movement. My palms rested on my thighs, and the fingers of my right hand were making small circles over top of the material of my pants. All of this—the rocking as well as the jean-based braille—was self-soothing, motions I'd seen my mother do often. My grandmother did it too. The hair on my arms stood on end when I realized it was me who was rocking.

My body gave Sara all the confirmation she needed. Bodies and brains are interesting that way, the first creating space for what the latter will eventually comprehend.

"Take a breath," she said, after I'd finished wiping the tears from my face.

"I'm okay," I said. "I'm okay."

I wasn't okay.

This wasn't a topic I'd ever pondered. What, exactly, did "bigger" mean in this context? Did I think I was better than my mother, more important? Did I think I was wiser in some way?

I would have answered no to all of those questions—a straight, cognitive no. But there's a limit to our cognition, a limit that our bodies, our somatic recognition, will stretch far beyond every time. Our minds don't have to know what a question means for our bodies to know the answer. And apparently, I knew the answer to this one in my bones. They told me so as they rattled.

I'd never really seen my mother, not all of her, not her in her totality. This realization, combined with the idea that her disappearance was already in motion, was too much to bear.

All of a sudden, everything I felt—my sadness, my smallness, my shame—came rushing forward. It moved through my hands like a great current. I wept, and as I did, I felt a last thread tear away. And from there, everything fell. Only, I wasn't sure what "everything" was. All I knew was the sensation—the feeling of a complete internal collapse.

"You need to remove the wall between you and your mother," said my therapist. "Whatever was built to keep you separate, needs to be taken down."

I wasn't sure what had been built, when, or even how it had been constructed—but the ripping I felt, the tearing away of some internal fabric was a sign that, whether I liked it or not, something was already happening.

The idea for the trip hit me almost as soon as the water did.

Go back to Montana, said a voice in my head as I stepped into the shower.

But I was just there, I thought.

I travel a fair bit, but I rarely, if ever, go back to places I've already been. Never mind places I've just returned from. And let me be clear: by "just," I mean that my luggage from a trip to Montana was still lying in the entryway of our house.

I grabbed the soap and brushed the idea aside. Not a minute later, it came back. Slightly altered this time.

Go back to Montana, I heard. *Take your mom with you.*

I paused before reaching for the shampoo.

Now that's interesting, I thought.

My mother and I had never really done things together, just the two of us. But given her recent Alzheimer's diagnosis, this seemed like a decent idea.

Maybe she needs something, I thought. *Maybe I'm supposed to help her with something.*

The idea that I might be in need of something never crossed my mind. Nor did the idea that she might be able to help me.

I rinsed myself off, got out of the shower, and forty minutes later I called my parents on a video chat.

I brought up the idea after a few minutes of small talk.

"Hey, Mom," I said. "The reason I'm calling is because I'm wondering if you might like to go on a trip with me."

She stared at me blankly and then looked at my dad.

I continued on.

"I was thinking we could take a road trip," I said. "Rent a car, drive through some national parks, maybe camp along the way."

"Do what?" she asked.

My mother was confused. It was hard for me to tell how much of this was because of the Alzheimer's or how much was because my mother found me to be a confusing person in general. We may not have had a track record of doing things together, but we did have a dossier of evidence regarding the frequency with which my decision-making confounded her.

"It's a road trip," I said. "In a car . . . with some camping. Just you and me."

"You and me?" she asked. "Where would we sleep?"

"We'd sleep in a tent," I said.

She looked back to my dad. In that moment, I wondered if she was seeking clarity, or permission, or perhaps just a safe place to hunker down.

I too looked at my dad. He was facing my mom, but I could see that his eyes were lit up. He knew this was a rare ask, and that if Alzheimer's wasn't part of our family's equation, perhaps this idea wouldn't be either.

"You'd sleep outside," he said to my mom before turning back to the camera. "She'd love to," he said.

"I would?" she asked, before quickly shrugging her shoulders and adding, "Well, okay. It sounds weird, but okay."

This was a sign of my mother's trust: her ability to surrender, to hand over the reins. As someone who regularly grasped for control, I found this trait difficult to understand.

My dad took the lead from there.

"When were you thinking of going?" he asked.

"As early as May," I said. "But . . . don't you have a golf trip to Scotland in June? What if we timed it around that?"

I watched as my dad's eyes lit up even more. It was perfect timing—he could go on his golf trip and not spend the whole time worrying about my mom, and she could come on a trip with me that I knew she would love.

My dad's response was instantaneous.

"Book it," he said with a smile.

And that's just what I did. I booked the trip, and then, because supplies would be needed, I promptly drove myself to REI.

Inside the store, I stopped in front of a locked display case full of things like Buck Knives and bear spray. I felt myself starting to sweat—first my armpits and then the palms of my hands.

Do I need these things? I wondered. *Should I be buying these things?*

I didn't know the answer to these questions because—wait for it—I'd never really been camping. I could count the number of nights I'd slept in a tent on two hands, and at least three of those occasions were sleepover parties spent in the Kerrisdale Wilderness (otherwise known as the manicured lawn in my parents' backyard). Most of the other occasions were at concert venues in my early twenties, where it was very likely that I was intoxicated. And while the final few times could be counted as actual camping, they occurred with friends who took care of the actual camping part. I honestly could not recount a time in my life, not ever, not once, where I'd built a fire, or lit a Jetboil stove, or pitched a tent by myself.

"I can do this," I whispered to myself, wiping my hands along the sides of my jeans. "We can do this."

All the while, I wasn't entirely sure what "this" was. Regardless, I felt called. Like whatever this was had been written in the stars, mapped out in advance by large constellations.

Three weeks later, my mother and I left for Montana—a place known for the vastness of its sky.

2

The Myth of an Ebb Tide

Nothing influences children more than the
silent facts in the background.

—CARL JUNG

I read a book once about mothers and daughters. It centered on the myth of Demeter and Persephone—about the dance between mothers and daughters, the natural cycle of daughters leaving and returning, going away and coming back home.

I loved the book, and at the same time I found it difficult to relate to the dance they described. My mother and I, I felt, had done no such dance. If there was a pattern to the way we moved through the world, it would be a simple tale about a tide that moved in one direction and a young woman who split off from herself to go with it—part of her moving out with the ocean, the other part remaining, sitting empty on the shore. This myth wouldn't include a return. It would be about that woman, that daughter, slipping out of herself and then ebbing for thirty-five years, moving ever outward, drawing lines in the sand as she went.

I drew my first when I was four years old. And the oddest thing about it was that my mother taught me how.

It happened in the stairwell of Marineview Preschool in Vancouver, British Columbia. The details are a patchwork in my brain, a first collection of images that weave together to form my earliest memory. My mother and I were standing together just inside the doorway of the preschool. There was a staircase that led up and another that led down. We were to take the latter.

"Down we go," my mom whispered, reaching out, suggesting I take her hand, which I did.

I used my other hand, my right hand, to grab the railing beside me, and together we moved slowly down the stairs, one big-girl step after another.

About halfway down I heard my mother's voice prompting.

"Say hello," she said softly.

I paused, looked up from my feet, and saw that there were two women standing at the bottom of the staircase, both of whom were smiling. I looked up at my mom. She nodded and smiled. I let go of the railing and offered a very timid wave.

One of the women waved back before moving up the staircase to greet us.

"Hi there," she said, as she crouched down in front of me. Her voice was singsongy and kind. She smelled like Play-Doh mixed with sugar and spice and everything nice.

"What's your name?" she asked.

I felt my mother's hand move. She rested it gently on my back.

"This is Stephanie," she said. "She's a little bit shy."

"Hi, Stephanie," said the lady in front of me. "I get shy too."

I looked up again at my mom.

"We've got her, Sheila."

This was the voice of the other lady, the one who still stood at the bottom of the stairs.

"It's just . . ." said my mom. "She . . ."

"We've got her," echoed the woman crouched in front of me. "We've done this a thousand times."

In that moment I felt a wave of worry move through my mother. I bobbed for a while inside of it. I knew this feeling. I was comforted by it. My mother's worry was a sign of her love. It was the steady hum of her, the white noise that ran in her background, something I could fall safely asleep to. I reached up, hoping to grab her hand again, but instead of taking it, instead of floating together in this wave of worry like we normally did, she bent over, put her hands on either side of my face, and gave me a big kiss on the cheek.

"You'll be fine," she whispered, not in a tone of confidence, but rather, hopeful persuasion. Her words were coated in concern. What she said didn't match what I sensed, what I knew she was feeling. It was the first time I remember feeling my mother move in two directions at once.

And then I watched as she turned herself around, made her way back up the stairs, and walked out the door. I was left on the staircase, swimming inside of her worry, which, in short order, had became my own.

Just before the door closed behind her, I collapsed onto the stairs and started to wail. My hands slapped on the rubber tread in protest. I screamed. The woman who had been crouching in front of me was now sitting beside me. Her arms were outstretched in an effort to comfort me. I smacked them away with ferocity, clumsily wiped at my face—my eyes, my nose, my wide, wailing mouth—and continued screaming. My hands became layered with dirt and dust as they moved back and forth from my wet, snotty face to the floor. To this day I hate having dirt on the palms of my hands.

When we went back the next day, I wore what my mother called "a brave face." Only it didn't feel brave. It felt like taking a droplet of my essence and flicking it from my fingertips. It felt like moving in two different directions at once.

Many things followed from those first days of preschool. Over time and a million unspoken lessons, I learned that although my mother felt things, she very rarely put those feelings into words. Instead, she chose action; she chose doing.

Her love was demonstrative and physical. You felt it in the way she hugged you and tucked you into bed. You tasted it in the cucumber sandwiches and the birthday cakes. You smelled it in the laundry. You knew she loved you simply because she was there.

I have many memories of being attached to my mother in a physical way. My arms wrapped around her waist in the morning. My face pressed up against the green velour robe she wore while filling the lunch bags we would carry off to school. Her fingers gently pulling through my wet summer hair as I sat curled up beside her on the dock—I used to watch the beads of sweat drip down her stomach before pooling in her belly button.

My mother gave me her physical body, but it seemed her emotional body was only partially there. While I can tell you what joy and contentment looked like on my mother's face, other emotions seemed to be missing—sorrow and grief, for example, as well as deep hurt. I cannot tell you what emotional pain looked like on the face of the woman who raised me.

I could feel these things as a fleeting undercurrent, but I couldn't see them on the surface of her. Words were absent too. There was no voice for her anger, no utterance of rage. My mother gave me many things, but candid conversation was not one of them. This was especially so when emotions were involved.

I came to understand that if my mother felt something uncomfortable, she simply moved away from it. She rolled inward. She busied herself, which was easy. There is, after all, a lengthy to-do list that comes with a family of six.

Through careful observation, I learned that nearly every feeling thing went without saying. These were the implicit rules for being a "big girl." This is what it meant to be strong. I understand now that it takes a certain kind of courage to feel and then give voice to one's discomfort. But growing up, as I watched those closest to me, I saw a different kind of courage, a courage of holding things in, of not naming things or speaking about them out loud, of storing them somewhere inside and moving in an alternate direction. My mother had this strength in spades. As did, it seemed, the rest of my family. A chatty bunch when it came to updating one another on the literal events of the day, but a bunch that used self-deprecation, sarcasm, and wit, or just plain silence about tender things, things like loneliness, sadness, anger, or despair.

I tried my best to mimic this familial fortitude, but I found it exhausting. This never-ending sensing and not saying was an onerous task for a feeling child, one who was also naturally talkative, obsessed with words and books and stories. Perhaps my love of words was born from desperation, from a deep desire for language with which to express a more complex range of emotions.

Once every month or so, this caused an implosion. On the days I felt overwhelmed by the feelings I had no words for, I would come home from school and quietly head to my room—the room where the ladybugs lived on the sill of the window. I would make sure the door was firmly closed behind me, and from there I would collapse on my bed in a long, moaning wail. I would cry for my mother over and over again—part of me desperate for her to come running with a basketfull of words to soothe me, to tell me what I was feeling and how to make sense of it all.

But there was another part of me, a bigger part that had already moved out with the tides. This was the part that had been flicking away droplets of my essence for weeks, months, years. I know this because as I screamed for my mother, I was also muffling my face with a pillow.

Simply put, I could not let her hear me. Somewhere inside of me, I knew it would have been more painful to have her sit beside me as I cried out for words—feeling part of her move toward me while another part rushed quickly away. To avoid all of this, it was me who moved, in a million different directions at once, searching madly for some shore I could land on, for some anchor and buoy I could latch on to and hold.

After the tears, I would fall into deep sleep, only to be woken for dinner. This happened with regularity from the ages of five to ten. And once I hit ten, I moved directly to the nap. There was no crying, no muffling. Just napping. Just a desire to have the inky black tide roll in and temporarily take me away.

If you see a child every day, it's almost impossible to notice them changing. You have to mark their height on the wall each year, or look at photos from each school year to convince yourself they've grown, to state with clarity that some significant change has occurred.

It's equally as hard to watch the ocean and notice it's ebbing. You have to commit the cycles of the moon to memory, or look carefully at the sand in order to be certain about which way the tides are swinging and what they're taking out to sea as they go.

It was difficult to understand the tipping point, to know when I had flicked too much of myself away. What day or month or year did it happen? When, officially, was there more of my essence on the outside of me than remained living inside?

There was nothing with which to measure the change. There was no doorjamb, no moon chart, no actual lines in the sand. It was all just a bunch of moments, blurred and bundled together. It was darn near impossible for anyone around me to add it all up, to connect all the dots. And with no vocabulary for this leaking of self, there was no chance for me to voice it, to give it a name.

By the time I was a teenager this practice was seamless—my emotional body moved out with the ocean, and my mental self remained on the shore. The ease with which I split off from my self was astounding. My naps turned into long sleeps, sometimes thirteen or fourteen hours at a time. I developed a deep suspicion of emotions. I questioned people who talked about them. I judged people who displayed them.

Why can't they keep it together? I would wonder in my head, not realizing I was the one who was splitting apart.

My family and the rest of the people around me lauded this performance—although it wasn't called a performance per se, but rather my personality. For the most part, I was calm and levelheaded. I was a sensible, confident young girl. My life was not dictated by a whirligig of teenage emotions, particularly the "female" kind.

I was valued for my pluck, for having the kind of motherly wit that my mother taught me, and I valued this myself. Albeit sometimes rebellious, I was mostly referred to as a good girl. This happened over and over again until I resigned myself to this collective definition. This is what a good girl was— performative, without even knowing there was a play going on or a script in my hand, without even seeing the curtains as they opened and closed.

As Sue Monk Kidd once wrote, "Once we are caught in the pattern of creating ourselves from cultural blueprints, it becomes a primary way of receiving validation."

It was so easy to convince the people around me that I was right there in front of them, when in fact, most of me was out on the ocean somewhere, treading water in a sea of roiling waves. And the person who was easiest to convince? The one hoodwinked by it all? Well, of course, that was me.

3

As Above, So Below

I watched my dad pull the car up to the curb at Vancouver International Airport. I saw him peer out the front windshield, looking around until he spotted me. He smiled and waved from inside the car. My mother was sitting in the passenger seat also scanning the area, looking like . . . well, like she didn't know what she should be looking for.

Based on my mother's Alzheimer's progression, meeting in Montana was out of the question. The plan was for me to fly into Vancouver, spend the night with my parents, and then fly with my mom into Bozeman. Our first stop would be Yellowstone National Park.

I motioned for my dad to pop the back gate of the car, and

as I loaded my bags I heard him giving a play-by-play to my mom.

"It's Steph," he said. "She's just arrived."

"Where?" she asked.

"Here," he said. "In Vancouver."

"But where's Steph?" she said, with a touch of frustration.

My dad pointed to the back of the open car.

"Right there. There she is," he said.

I waved, but my mom wasn't looking. Something in the conversation had hooked onto the synapses inside of her brain.

"We're in Vancouver?" she asked, her voice thick with confusion.

How am I supposed to see her as bigger when she is in the midst of disappearing? I thought to myself.

I closed the back gate of the car and took a deep breath. In the handful of weeks since seeing my therapist, I had thought about the promise I'd made, about removing whatever had been built between my mother and me, about seeing her whole. But in this moment, all I could see were the things that were missing. It had only been eleven months since her diagnosis, and yet there was already so much less of her.

I opened the side door of the car and slid into the back seat.

"Hi, Mom!" I said.

It was almost as if you could hear her brain click into gear.

"Oh, I was wondering if that was you!" she said, reaching her hand back to squeeze mine. "You look different. Your hair is so much longer. And darker! When did your hair get so dark?" she asked.

I didn't look different. My hair was not so much longer.

Nor was it anything other than my standard shade of chocolate brown. My mother's memory of me was shifting. I decided, in that moment, to shift with it.

"Really?" I asked, pulling a section of my hair forward for examination. "Maybe it's gotten a bit darker this winter."

"I think so," she said. "It's so much darker. It looks pretty."

She squeezed my hand one more time before continuing on. "Are you just here for the night?" she asked.

"No, Mom," I said. "We're going on a trip together. I'm in town to pick you up."

"We are?" she asked. "You are?"

My dad interjected, "She . . . you and Steph are going camping. Remember? We've been talking about it. And we've been packing."

I caught my dad's eye as he was glancing back at me in the rearview mirror.

"We started laying a few things out," he said. "But I thought you could help."

"I sure can," I said, completely glossing over my concern about just how short-term her short-term memory had gotten. I knew she was beginning to lose things that had happened a month back or even a week prior, but this seemed worse. She didn't even remember the trip they'd been so recently talking about—a trip that just yesterday, or perhaps that morning, she had started packing for.

This was the new pattern with my mom—a sort of guessing game about her progression, about who she was and where she was in any given moment, about how much she had lost, and what parts of her were left.

And although my father had said it, I was doubtful she needed help packing. This was, after all, the woman who had spent a lifetime making all things luggage look like a competitive sport—knowing what six people and a slobbering dog would need when traveling, and then being able to jigsaw two weeks' worth of those items, plus food, water skis, and life jackets, into the back of a VW van before the rise of roof racks.

As it turned out, I was wrong. She did need help with the packing. When we got to the house, I saw that a pair of red jeans, two white cotton turtlenecks, and a red zip-up sweater had been placed on top of the dresser. Beside them were a pair of turquoise, knee-length shorts, black leggings, and a grey wrap.

We repacked. Although she would not relent on the turtlenecks, nor the grey wrap.

"What if I get cold?" she asked, over and over.

"Right," I said, faking agreement. "Good point."

I had learned enough in the eleven months since her diagnosis to know that arguing with a person who has Alzheimer's is as useless as . . . well, as a thin cotton turtleneck in the mountains of Montana. I snuck as much wool clothing into her bag as I could find, as well as a down jacket and vest, before zipping it closed.

After that, I walked down the hall, toward the room where the ladybugs still lived on the sill of the window. This was my childhood home, a place that felt more familiar to me than even my self did—and yet, in that moment, nothing felt familiar. I climbed into the same bed I'd slept in when I was a child, just down the hall from my mother, who in so many ways felt nothing like my mother at all.

What if our story is like Demeter and Persephone's? I wondered to myself. *Only in our version, when Persephone finally returns, she discovers her mother all but gone? What happens then?*

Over the past handful of hours I had become filled with doubt that this trip would show me who my mother was. I wondered if I might be too late, if too many shafts and shutters of memory had already closed, if too much was already missing.

This felt overwhelming to me. But the overwhelm didn't last very long, for one familiar thing did end up happening that night. The inky black water flowed in, and I was asleep underneath it before my head hit my childhood pillow.

"I've never done this before," my mother announced with excitement as we stood checking in for our flight.

This, of course, was not true. For the last thirty or forty years, my mother traveled on planes a minimum of once or twice a year. But it wasn't a lie either. How could it be when no memory of those travels existed in her head? It was somewhere in between. In a lost place. This is what Alzheimer's is—a watery confluence of neither here nor there.

"I feel like I'm a little kid," she added before turning and looking directly at the woman behind the counter. "I have no idea how any of this works."

The woman behind the counter looked over to me, her face saying what most people's faces had begun to say when interacting with my mother: *Something's a little off here but I can't quite put my finger on it.*

It makes sense, really. What is a person supposed to make of a woman who appears quite put together, who seems Jane Fonda fit, but who is, at the very same time, making statements only a time traveler would?

I smiled at the woman and then turned to my mom, resting my hand gently on her back.

"I'll show you how it all works," I said.

"You know how all of this works?!" she replied. She was dumbfounded . . . and then, very quickly, relieved.

"Yep," I said. "You just relax."

Once we were checked in for our flight, I steered my mother through security and toward a wine bar near our gate, where I promptly ordered us each a glass of champagne. She talked the entire time. She asked lots of questions, made a variety of interesting observations, and then asked some more questions. It was not unlike spending time with a well-mannered nine-year-old who had been oversaturated in curiosity.

"This one?" she asked, pointing to one of the barstools. "Are you sure? Where are you going to sit?"

"I'll sit right here," I said, pulling out the barstool next to hers.

"Oh, there's another one. Well that worked out well, didn't it?"

The bartender placed her drink in front of her.

"Is this for me?" she whispered, reluctant to take the drink. "I don't have my wallet."

"I've got my wallet, Mom. Don't worry."

"You do?" she asked. "Shouldn't I have mine? Where's my purse?"

"Right there," I said. Her purse was resting in her lap, the strap of it still across her body.

"Well that's a good place for it," she said with a laugh, before pointing back to her glass of champagne. "So I can have this?" she asked. "Where's yours?"

"I've got mine right here," I said.

"Oh . . ." she said, looking over to my glass. "I'm not a fussy person. So you could have had this one, but we both have one, so that's good."

We raised our glasses in the air.

"Cheers!" she said, putting one of her arms around me. "To . . ."

She paused.

Was she searching for the right word, I wondered, or was she confused about who, exactly, I was?

"To mothers and daughters!" I said, filling in the blank, before clinking our glasses together.

"Where's Brian?" she asked, after taking a sip of her drink.

"He's at home. It's just you and me on this trip."

"He's not coming?"

"Nope. Just you and me . . . we're going camping."

"We are?"

She thought about that for a while, and as she did, I watched a bit of worry snake up to the surface of her.

"Do we have everything we need for that?" she asked.

"We sure do," I said.

"Okay. I was just wondering."

She took another sip of her champagne and then looked back to me.

"What do we need for that? Did you say we're going tenting?"

"Don't worry about it, Mom. I packed everything we need. Just enjoy your drink."

When it came time to pay, I tucked some money into the check presenter, stood up, and began gathering our things.

"Okay, Mom," I said. "Grab that bag. It's time to go."

"But you can't just leave that there," she said, pointing at the check presenter.

I was already moving away from the bar, but she stayed standing next to the stools.

"Come on, Mom," I said.

"You're just going to leave that there?"

She was cringing.

"The bartender knows," I said in frustration. "It's okay."

"He knows . . . are you sure?" She was inching away from the bar, reluctant to leave money just sitting there.

"I'm sure," I said firmly.

I grabbed her hand and began to tug her along. "Time to go, Mom," I said.

Her eyes were glued to the check presenter. "Bu—Oh. Oh, he just took it. Okay. We can go."

She smiled at me and squeezed my hand.

"Where are we going?" she asked.

I didn't answer.

My mother's brain is like a tangled gold chain. Delicate links that move this way and that are now all balled up in a knot. And I am just beginning to learn that no matter how hard I try, no matter how much patience I give it, nor how many jewelers are brought in to examine it, with their expert hands and tiny pins, the chain will never come undone.

The boarding area was bustling with activity. We stood off to the side and I began pulling our passports out of my bag. Once I had everything sorted, I looked up at the prompter to see if they had begun calling any boarding zones. Thirty or forty seconds passed without a single comment or question from my mother, so I turned to make sure she was still standing beside me. She was right there, quietly looking around at all the people, rocking gently on her feet. It was a subtle heel-to-toe movement. We were both doing it—back and forth, back and forth, back and forth.

I remembered us standing together just like that only a few weeks before.

My mother's mother had died on January 30 of that year. She was cremated five days later, and on Mother's Day, a day prior to what would have been her ninety-sixth birthday, my family gathered in Vancouver for her wake.

That morning, I helped my mom decide what to wear. And that afternoon, I walked with her into a room full of our family—siblings, aunts, uncles, and cousins. Of the blood relatives in the room, there were twenty-one women and ten men.

How have I never noticed this before? I thought to myself, taking in the wellspring of women around me.

As we entered, I could sense my mother's nerves. We stood together near a window at the edge of the room. She leaned slightly into me and both of us rocked—heel to toe, heel to toe.

"I don't know any of these people," she said quietly. Her concern was heavy.

This, of course, was not true. She knew she was supposed to know them, and yet, she didn't. It was another watery confluence.

"Look at how many people there are." She continued, "I just . . . I just don't know any of them. I haven't seen them in thirty years."

I didn't correct her. It seemed a cruel thing to do in the midst of her mother's funeral service.

After some time, she turned to me in excitement. The confusion had lifted, and her eyes were suddenly hopeful.

"Is my mom coming?" she asked.

The question cast a stone straight through me. I felt it skip and land at the base of my throat. I swallowed.

"No, Mom," I said, looking at her soft, smiling face. "Granny's not coming."

She looked back at me. I watched her smile slowly collapse, air seeping from the edges of her mouth.

"I knew that already, didn't I?" she asked.

"Yes," I said. "You did."

"I've known that for months, haven't I?" she asked.

"Yes," I said. "You have."

Although she remained unmoved, standing beside me, I felt some part of her fall. I sensed a crumpling, as if some invisible part of my mother was now lying on the ground inside of herself.

Is she sad? I wondered as I reached for her hand. *Is this her sadness?*

I knew there would be no words, especially now, especially with the Alzheimer's. To understand what was happening I had to feel it, I had to sense it and fill any gaps with a rough translation. It's what I'd always had to do.

I'm not sure what my mother needed from her mother. I had never asked, and she had never told me. But in that moment, I understood that she too had learned to split off from herself. I watched her forget and then remember that her mother was gone, realize and then re-realize that she had no person to return to, no shore to call home, and I felt it. The way she held herself together at the same time as letting a part of herself go. The way she sat and waited for a wave to come and carry her out to sea. I knew that feeling. I knew it well.

Had my mother cried alone in her bedroom? Were we both lost at sea? Rocking gently in a boat somewhere—back and forth, back and forth, back and forth.

Perhaps we were more alike than I thought—a notion that was both comforting to me and completely unbearable.

A few days after my grandmother's wake, a smaller group of family, including my mother's three sisters—Daphne, Brenda, and Nancy—were gathered in a garden at St. Mary's Anglican for the internment of her ashes.

I remember staring at the minister's shoes. They were too casual. They were nonslip sneakers. They were the kind of shoe a TSA agent would wear as they sifted through luggage with blue rubber gloves on. Up until that point, I'd never considered what was or was not appropriate footwear for a minister, but these shoes were not it. Faded black sneakers aren't meant to be worn whilst handling an urn, nor the grief of the family attached to it.

My eyes moved from the minister's shoes to the small hole in the ground. It had been dug before we arrived and wasn't big enough for anything more than a sapling. But that's not what we were planting. The minister said a few words, as well as a short prayer, and then he poured my grandmother's ashes into the small hole.

The ashes slid out of the urn and I heard them as they hit the bottom of the hole. It was the sound a quart of flour would make if you poured it into a large wooden bowl. A puff of ash wafted up. That was it. That was my grandmother. A mighty oak burned down and poured into a hole made for a sapling. I linked my arm through my mother's beside me.

I looked down at our feet. We were rocking yet again. This wasn't something we had to remember to do. It was autonomic. It was knowledge that lived inside of us, memory attached to our muscles.

Something inside of us knew how to do this. Something that had no name and no words.

I felt a pull somewhere inside of me.

Is this the language we share? I wondered to myself.

As a little girl, I used to play a game with my grandmother whenever she was visiting. I would ask my mom to sit beside her, and then I'd say, "Hands, please."

They knew the drill. They would each hold out one hand, side by side in the air. I would line mine up next to my mom's, and then, one by one, I'd pinch the tops of our hands. I would grab a little bit of skin, pull it up as gently as I could, and then let go. From there, we would giggle together as we watched the skin, carefully observing how it moved back into place. Mine snapped back with youthful elasticity. My mom's slowly melted toward her hand. And my grandmother's, for the most part, stayed where I'd pulled it—like a miniature mountain range running from her knuckles straight down to her wrist. She had to massage it, adding a little warmth to her papery skin to make it go back to normal.

This image is carved in my memory. Every time I see a ridgeline in the distance I think of my grandmother's hands. But I don't know how long the carving will last.

My grandmother had dementia.

My mother has Alzheimer's.

I am a sapling inside of a forest that seems hell-bent on forgetting.

As a young girl, I didn't see myself like them, and now, I don't want to be like them. I don't want to be planted in this soil, rooted in what seems to be scorched earth, burned in a fire of forgetfulness. But here I am, full of quaking fear that the phrase "as above, so below" runs also in the opposite direction. That the groundwater running through my lineage is poisoning the bloodline—that it runs from our roots, all the way into our brains.

It terrifies me to think I am living inside an inheritance of unspoken emotion, of minds that eventually cave in on themselves. What a farce it is—the perception of safety we've created by living almost entirely inside of our heads. When I think about my DNA holding on to a memory about how to forget, something inside of me falls silent, goes numb. I do not know how to name what it is, nor how to dig it up and out. So I just sit. I petrify. I let that part turn into stone.

Do I have three decades or four? I wonder to myself.

My body was born with instructions about how to walk, and how to talk, and how to transform from a child into a woman. Instructions that came with a timer built in. Would this knowledge of how to forget work the same way?

I remember reading a line from Joy Harjo's book *Crazy Brave.* "Bones have consciousness," she wrote. "Within marrow is memory." These words made something inside of me pant.

When will the bomb go off? I ask inside my head. *What day is the timer set for, the one that will trigger the instructions about how to forget?*

In that moment in St. Mary's garden, and in many other moments since, I've thought about the elasticity of my memory, about when it will begin to fade as my mother's and grandmother's did, and about how and where my brain will begin losing itself. And I worry that, as a collective, when you line up the women in my family one after the next, we will begin to form a mountain range of forgetfulness, creating a series of abstracted ridgelines that run clear across our ancestral landscape.

The thought of this torments me. Because what happens when a lineage of women forget themselves? Who do the daughters return to when they can't remember who they are? What mothers will exist for us then? Who will hold us in the midst of our collapse?

This felt like a curse, like Persephone lost forevermore in the underworld, and Demeter with no daughter to find—a lost destiny, an irretrievable ancestry. These questions hung in the air around me as my mother and I flew from Vancouver to Bozeman.

Our flight went directly over the Rocky Mountains, a colossal divide that sweeps down from British Columbia and Alberta into Idaho, Wyoming, Montana, and beyond. And as I sat on the plane, gazing at the massive ridgeline below, I felt the energy of the natural world flood into my body.

Maybe it's this, I thought to myself, taking a deep breath as my mother dozed in the seat beside me. *Maybe this is what I can return to. And maybe, if my mother did split off from herself, maybe she can return here too.*

This was not the first time I had run to Mother Nature looking for guidance. She had been a source of wisdom for me many times in the past, a provenance of hard-edged veracity that, with enough time, melted into solace. The very best part about being in nature is that the truth meets you there, which is also the reason it's hardest to go. At the same time, I was hopeful about this trip, about Mother Nature yielding wisdom yet again. About the idea that I might find some answers here in the Rockies—a ridgeline so long it has a chance to connect our past to our present to our future. Perhaps the answers were somewhere inside these gargantuan folds, tucked amongst the mountains and lakes, the rocks and rivers and streams.

For a brief moment in time, this trip made sense to me—as Alzheimer's stole words and whole phrases, an entire language of memory, it seemed like we were being presented with the opportunity to learn a new one, or recover a lost one. I held on to the idea that Mother Nature might be able to bring us both back to shore.

All of the questions I had about the splitting off from ourselves, as well as how we might find our way back to wholeness, were momentarily quelled. Because if there is anything, any person or any place, that will remember us all—when the root rot sets in, when our synapses, each and every one of them, no longer fire—it has to be Mother Nature. She had to be the one who remembered, just as the skin on my grandmother's hands did.

4

Pray, Montana

*The way we deal with loss shapes our capacity
to be present to life more than anything else.
The way we protect ourselves from loss may
be the way in which we distance ourselves
from life.*

—RACHEL NAOMI REMEN

My mother and I arrived in Bozeman on June 6. We deplaned, picked up our luggage, and walked over to the rental car desks.

"I've never done this before," my mother announced with excitement as we stood waiting for the attendant to hand us the keys to our car.

This, of course, was not true. But what is truth anyway?

We stayed at a small Airbnb that night, and we laughed over pizza and beer. That felt like truth.

But will it stay that way, I thought, *or will it slip into the arena of a lie when she doesn't remember any of it the very next day?*

In the morning, we went to the grocery store to stock up

on oatmeal and eggs, apples and Babybel cheese. We got some coffee and a few cans of Campbell's tomato rice soup. My mother loved that soup. That felt like truth—but was it truth if I had to remind her of it?

At about ten in the morning we drove out of Bozeman and made a quick stop at a small bookstore in a town called Livingston. I bought a postcard for my grandmother, something I'd always done when I traveled. She had been gone for close to six months, but I felt like I had to buy one anyway.

This, I thought to myself. *This is truth.* But even then I wasn't sure.

We drove down the stretch of road that runs from Pray, Montana, to the northern entrance of Yellowstone, the road that runs all the way to Boiling River. Otherwise known as Paradise Valley. A handful of miles in, I watched a spell come over my mother. I knew it took place because I watched my mother's face as it cracked wide open and burst into tears. She cried her way through that whole stretch of road on the morning we drove it. A levee, one I never knew existed inside of her, broke clean away.

Have you ever been to a place that cast a spell on you? A place that sent a mesmerizing spark, a scattershot of luminescence, flying through the air and right on into your bloodstream? I've been to a few of these places, but Yellowstone National Park stands out as the most magical. The most potent of portals.

For me it has something to do with the bison. They look like an answer to a prayer. Like if a person was crying and alone and they asked God to send them something or someone who understood, I think she might send a bison, or perhaps a whole herd. Something that would help them run into the storm, through the clouds and the driving rain, through the electricity of it all, clear to the other side. I think, perhaps, that's what I had been doing all those years in my bedroom. I think I'd been praying for bison.

There's something prehistoric about them—like they come from a time and a place where the heartbeat of everything around us could be heard, could be felt through hooves that pounded the earth.

Every time I see a herd of bison it throws me back in time and flips me forward at once—like I've been hit with some sort of reminder, an omen that I need to watch what I carry, and I need to watch what carries me. Every time I see a bison, I am reminded that it is okay to be the one who runs into the storm.

My mother cried something fierce that morning on the road. So much so, I finally pulled the car off to the side.

"Mom?" I asked. "What's happening?"

I was genuinely concerned she was hurt in some way.

"Are you okay?" I went on. "Why are you crying?"

Nerves bounced up and down in my body. I wasn't sure what to do, nor how or who to be in this moment with her.

"Mom?!" I asked again.

It took her some time to find her voice, but when she did, she said three careful words:

"It's so beautiful."

I felt suddenly calm. I didn't know a lifetime of thirst could be slaked with three words. I grabbed her hand and sat back in my seat. We stared out the window at the river valley brushed out before us, the mountains rising up in every direction. It was, using Annie Dillard's words, "an infinite storm of beauty."

Emigrant Peak and the rest of the Absaroka Mountains climbed up to the east and the Gallatin Range up to the west. We were held in this place in between. It was a cradle, a womb made of river water and stone. And even though I couldn't see it, I knew there was a great thaw occurring right there in front of us. Somewhere in those mountains the snow was melting; huge volumes of water were tumbling down from the peaks, rushing right into the creeks and streams that feed the Yellowstone River. A thaw like that can be painful at first. An aching pulse that beats inside your fingertips.

"Look," she said, as if she'd never laid eyes on a river valley or been anchored somewhere in the mountains. "Look at all this nature."

And with that simple incantation, the spell for our entire trip was cast. This was my mother in nature. This was Mother Nature. This was my mother's nature. I'd seen them on their own, but I'd never really witnessed them partner together. Not like this.

My mother took a hitched breath in and let a long sigh out. A sign she was ready to keep going. I checked for traffic and slowly pulled the car back onto the road. About six or seven miles later, I felt my mother lean slightly in toward my right shoulder.

"I've been here before," she whispered.

This, of course, was not true. But who was I to say who

my mother was, what her truth was, where she had or had not been?

I didn't know very many answers when it came to my mother. I didn't know very many questions either. Everything I had ever done, every choice I'd ever made, had been a desperate attempt to prove I didn't need anything from my mother. My swift move in the opposite direction, the sizeable ego I'd built up around our differences—all of it, my entire life, had been fabricated using the following mantra, the subconscious stitching that said: I will not become my mother.

How many times had I whispered these words, or some variation of them, to my friends: "Oh god, I'm turning into her, aren't I? Please don't let me turn into my mother."

How many times had my sister and I rolled our eyes together before saying, "Stop. That is so Mom. Stop right now." You can't. How many times had I disagreed with people when they told me I looked like my mom, was like my mom, or reminded them of her in any way?

"Really?" I'd ask. "I don't see it." And I didn't. This wasn't a lie. No evidence of our similarities existed in my head.

Inside all of this had been an unconscious but forceful shove. A rejection that ran so deep it became seamless, invisible even to me. What a mysterious thing it is, to reject some part of yourself with such ferocity that you genuinely no longer see it. And perhaps even more so, that you forget it even exists.

As we drove through the rest of the valley, I realized that I'd never known the answers to the questions about who my mother really was. The wholeness of her truth had been evasive, was felt fleetingly. Was that because she didn't want to be known, or because I'd pushed her away? Was it because some piece had gone missing? Was it because she didn't know her whole self and thus couldn't share it—verbally or otherwise? I didn't know. I wasn't sure. Some things are so easy to be sure about; others . . . others feel like a watery confluence.

I am asked a fair number of questions about my mother and her Alzheimer's, but there is one question that stands out from the bunch, one question that is asked the most.

"How did you know?" they ask. "I mean, how did you know for sure?"

This question is not being asked in curiosity's tone, nor for curiosity's sake.

There are currently 5.8 million people in America living with Alzheimer's. According to the Alzheimer's Association, another person in the United States develops the disease every 65 seconds.

The question I get about my mother isn't actually a question, but rather, a begging. People are pleading for something not to be true. Just underneath the queries, I hear whispered voices slipping through.

"Dear God," I hear them say. "Please not her. Please not him. Please not us."

I know all of this because that's what we were saying too.

I don't remember my mother being diagnosed. I don't remember receiving the news, or if it came by way of a somber phone call or an emotional email. Obviously, it happened, and common sense tells me I would have heard the news from my father, but I don't remember for sure. None of the days or weeks soaked up by the summer of 2015 stand out in my mind as important markers in our family's Alzheimer's story arc. I know this sounds insensitive—like how is it possible that I can recall the exact place in which I stood, as well as the feeling of my fingertips gently circling over top of my maroon-colored skirt, when the news broke about the death of Princess Diana, but I can't pull up a single thread of memory about the moment I was told my mother had Alzheimer's?

My answer to that, if it is in fact a question, is this—*I already knew.*

Alzheimer's doesn't just appear out of nowhere; it's not a surprise-party kind of disease. There are signs. It's a slow and steady build. It's like the family of mice that are currently living somewhere inside the walls of our kitchen. I was not surprised when we caught the first one. That wasn't the moment I announced, "We have mice!" I knew it months prior to the first snap of the trap.

It started with wondering. The temperatures had dropped low enough to warrant some heat, and about an hour after turning the thermostat up I smelled something funny. Weeks later, I thought about it briefly when I noticed a small hole in the plywood behind the kitchen sink. And I considered it a possibility when we found two traps in the pantry, set by the previous owners of the house. But it was well into winter before I added it all up, before I voiced what I already knew to be true. "We have mice," I said, when we came home to a spilling of small, black droppings close to the garbage can—the one that lived under the sink, with the mice, obviously.

It took months, and visible mouse shit, before I allowed myself to be certain, before I called the truth the truth.

This is how it was with my mother's Alzheimer's. The diagnosis itself wasn't shocking or traumatic for me. It was as obvious as the mice—the evidence was everywhere. Little pieces of it were being placed in front of me, one after another, begging me to take on the role of Miss Marple in an Agatha Christie play about things going missing in my mother's brain.

Evidence was being dropped for all of us, but evidence like that isn't something we're excited to find. More often than not we ignore these small clues. We turn the other way, we convince ourselves we didn't see what we saw, we ignore it, we script it into a different story, and we tell ourselves there is some other, very good, totally explicable reason for the signs we are seeing.

"Half of being in a family is just ignoring stuff," said author Omar El Akkad, and my family . . . we lived this.

"She's been stressed about Granny. Once Granny's in the care home, Mom will relax."

"Look, she's never been good with names. Give her a break."

"Remember that time she typed a whole email into the subject line because she didn't know how to move the cursor into the body of the email—she never learned how to use email on the computer, never mind email on her phone. Get off her back."

"She's in her sixties, of course she's going to forget a word here or there. Leave her alone."

The last bits of those sentences—that was how I knew.

Anytime something surfaced, the collective response was something like, "Leave her alone."

But the truth is—we weren't saying, "Leave my mother alone." We were saying, "Leave me alone." We were saying, "I'm scared," and "I don't want this to be true," and "I won't be able to handle it if it is." We were begging, "Please not her. Please not us. Please not this."

When every person around you is saying they're scared, albeit in some coded way, chances are high of there being scary things in the midst. And when every person around you is already begging, albeit veiled in avoidance and covered over in questions, chances are you all know what the scary thing is.

My mother was thirty-two years old when she sensed that parts of me were being formed. She was thirty-three when she felt it for certain, when she knew it in her bones.

I was thirty-two years old when I sensed that pieces of my mother were going missing, when I sensed that little bits of her were slipping through cracks in her brain. I was thirty-three when I felt it for certain, when I knew it in my bones.

When people ask me how I knew, they lay down bread crumbs, small clues that center around lost words, and names not remembered, and unpredictable outbursts of anger. They talk about forgetfulness, and repetition, and the need for constant reminders. They say, "She says things now that she would never have said in the past." Or, "Yesterday, he got confused about the streetlights." When people present me with all of the evidence, it tells me they already know. Somewhere inside, they know the truth. They are racking their brains for the answers when their bones have known the real story for some time. They are rocking back and forth, back and forth, back and forth—not sure anymore about how to be sure, not wanting what's true to be true.

A lot can happen when we wait for our brains to catch up. A lot can occur between the moment we smell the mice and the moment we say, "They are here. There is something living inside of the walls."

From a very young age I understood that you're not supposed to tell the truth. I mean, you're not supposed to lie either . . . but also, don't tell the truth. And don't give voice to what you think might be the truth. Oh, also, don't even make a suggestion. It's better that way. *Just be agreeable,* they said without saying, *and nonconfrontational.* Those are more "likable" things.

I wasn't able to keep what I knew about my mother on the inside. I didn't carry enough of that particular familial strength to keep my thoughts to myself. I wasn't able to feel one thing and do another, know something and say nothing. I couldn't do it anymore. Not that I'd done a great job of it to begin with.

So I did what my family would wordlessly call "crossing the line." I ran to my father and I ran to my mother. I collected the clues and the puzzle pieces and the evidence that had gathered all around us and placed it gently in front of them. And then I watched as both of them covered their eyes. It was too hard a thing to look at.

I ran next to my sister, and I placed all that I saw at her feet. "Look," I said. "Do you see this? Tell me you see this too."

She paused. Long enough for the skin on my grandmother's hands to settle back into place.

"Yes," she said. "I see it. I've been seeing it for a year."

Part of me stood standing. Another part of me fell to the floor.

Has my sister been crying alone in her bedroom?

There was no comfort in this. The only thing this was was unbearable.

Did all of the women in my family keep things inside of themselves—away from others? What else did we know and not say? What else did we feel and not give voice to? Were we all, each and every one of us, splitting off from ourselves, drowning out the voices of our sadness and fear with ebbs of salt water? Were we all using shame to muffle the sound of our cries?

Ever since my mother's diagnosis, I had been consumed by the idea that what was coded in my grandmother had been coded in my mother, and was, at birth, also coded in me. That I too would be swallowed whole by the gaps and pits and crevices destined to form in my brain, as would the other women around me—my aunts, my sister, my cousins and nieces.

But now, it seemed none of this mattered. Pushed aside was the great looming fear of a genetic predisposition to forget. In its place was a trembling sense that we might be hollow already, that a whole group of us might have learned, generation after generation, to split off from ourselves, from the sanctity of our anger, from the whole truth of who we are.

Because what does forgetting one's self even matter if you can't recall what wholeness feels like in the first place? Who would teach us how to come back to ourselves, if the only lessons we knew were how to move away? After lifetimes of dismembering ourselves, how could we expect to re-member?

This wasn't about pulling up the roots of Alzheimer's to see where and how they might be connected to me. This was about examining the very soil we'd been planted in.

I wonder if it is possible for a singular feeling to lodge itself so far into the bone that we shape the rest of our lives around it. And if that feeling made its way into the marrow, would all our daughters to come shape their lives around it as well?

It took my sister and me another year to convince my dad to take my mother to the doctor. For him to take her. Because by that time, she was too far gone to take herself. That's how long we waited. My whole family holding my mother in our arms—rocking back and forth, back and forth, trying to find a way to move from unconscious despair to the searing pain of conscious grief, trying to figure out how to give words to the things we were sensing but had learned no language for.

It's what taught me the difference between begging and praying.

Begging is what you do when you sense something scary is true. Praying is what you do when you're driving through a river valley, trying to find a way to turn all that fear into some sort of surrender.

5

Little White Lies

After lunch that first day we stopped at a convenience store in Gardiner, a small town–cum–adventure outfitter that borders Yellowstone National Park. I had forgotten to buy cream at the grocery store in Bozeman, and we also needed ice and a bundle or two of firewood.

I opened the door to the shop and heard a small bell jingle above us. We stepped in, and as I looked around to get my bearings, I felt my mom's arm slide into the crook of mine. We walked down an aisle toward the dairy section, and as my mom scanned the shelves, she shrieked.

"Oh!" she said. "This is a liquor store too!"

Convenience stores in Canada don't sell liquor.

"I want to see if they have that drink I like," she continued.
She paused for a moment and turned to me.

"What is that drink I like?" she asked.

"It's Glayva, Mom. You like Glayva."

All of this was a bit surprising to me, as my mom had never been much of a drinker. Every now and again my dad would pour her an ounce or two of Glayva—a sweet whiskey liqueur—or perhaps a glass of prosecco. I have a handful of memories of seeing my mother slightly tipsy at a wedding or special occasion—the dead giveaway being a bouncy shoulder dance that her eyebrows cannot help but accompany—but that said, I'd never seen her drunk.

Yet since her diagnosis, a nightcap or three seemed both routine and harmless. I wasn't sure why her drinking had increased. Maybe it was to numb. Maybe it was to let loose after a lifetime of keeping it together. Maybe there was no reason at all.

"Are you sure?" she asked me.

"Yep," I replied. "But . . ."

I paused. I knew a bottle of Glayva would be an unlikely find at a convenience store, but I thought there might be a decent alternative. I looked around to see row after row of Bud Light before coming across a small section that was full of Jack Daniel's, Fireball, and various types of Bacardi.

"I don't think they're going to have it here, Mom."

"Well, let's see," she said as she began scouring the shelves. She was oddly intent.

She proceeded to march up and down the aisles holding up random bottles as she went. "Is this it?" she would ask.

"Nope. Not that," I would say.

"What about this? Are you sure it wasn't that last one? That looked familiar to me."

"No. Not that one."

My mother must have picked up about nine or ten bottles before I spotted a shelf full of Baileys. Not Glayva, but something I knew she would like.

"This one, Mom! Here it is."

"Are you sure?" she asked. "That doesn't look like it."

"This is it," I said firmly, as I put the bottle in the cart.

I didn't want to play the guessing game anymore. And I didn't want to stop and explain that this was a small convenience store and not a full liquor store like the ones they have in Canada, so it probably wouldn't have Glayva. I didn't want to answer questions about Glayva. I also didn't want to answer questions about the thousand other bottles of booze on the shelf. I didn't want to explain to her what Baileys was, and that no, it wasn't Glayva, but yes, she had tried it on multiple occasions, and also yes, she had quite liked it over ice, and that's why we needed the ice . . . so could we just put the bottle in the cart and go get ice. I didn't want to move slowly. I didn't want to mother my mother.

I walked over to the large freezer. She followed me. She stood silently behind me as I grabbed a few bags of ice. She waited quietly as I placed them in the cart. She followed behind me again as we made our way to the firewood. Once we were there she grabbed the bottle of Baileys out of the cart.

"How do you know this is it?" she asked. Her voice was laced with a blend of suspicion and frustration.

"I just know," I said, grabbing the bottle out of her hand and placing it back in the cart.

She didn't have the words for it, but she knew I wasn't telling all of the truth.

When did this become a regular thing? I wondered. The fibs, the little white lies, my hands grabbing for small pieces of wool to pull up and over my mother's eyes, all so I could move a little quicker, all to make it just a little bit easier. I thought it was harmless. I thought she wouldn't notice. But some part of her did.

It's fairly common practice to lie to a person with Alzheimer's or those with other forms of dementia. In the beginning, when they mix things up or get confused, your first instinct is to correct them.

"No, Mom. We're not in Vancouver today, we're in Montana."

"No, Mom. Yesterday wasn't the day we flew on the plane, that was earlier this week."

But those corrections usually lead to small disagreements. These short-lived back-and-forths would be frustrating and almost always end in confusion, in my mother scouring her brain for information that fit the reality I was talking about, as opposed to the one she could swear was occurring.

One learns, rather quickly, to fib, to bend reality to fit that of the person with the disease. I found this easy. It wasn't too far a leap from my early lessons in "truth-telling," the notion that you should be agreeable and nonconfrontational, that you should never say too much, but rather just enough.

"It *has* been a long time since you've been camping. Ages, really." After we had camped the night prior.

"I know. Isn't it delicious? It's called oatmeal." After she claimed she had never tasted such a thing in her life.

"Yes. You're right. I think you do know that woman from school." After walking by a complete stranger thirty years her junior at the Bozeman airport.

But there were bigger lies too, lies that carried more weight, ones that felt like a larger betrayal of truth.

"Yes. Sisters! Just two sisters on a camping trip."

"Oh, you don't have to worry about your kids. They're at home with Brian. I bet they're playing in the backyard."

These were lies that required I also lie to myself. They ushered me into a place where I had to deny bigger things, like my own feelings and parts of my identity. This too was relatively easy, for a certain economy of truth had also been woven into my inheritance of being. Words, even when they were few and far between, often spoke louder than actions, louder than the energy I sensed was hovering in the air.

Ever since I was little I can remember having a strong sense about other people's emotions, even if I couldn't name them. But when I asked, when I searched for external confirmation about whether my body was sensing the truth, I was nearly always told no. And this is the most duplicitous and confusing lie of them all—an emotional subterfuge, a lesson in how your body is deceiving you.

"Are you sad?" I would ask, sensing a faucet dripping slowly inside someone's body.

"No," they would say. "Why would I be sad?"

"Are you mad?" I would mumble, picking up on the

tightness inside of my mother, as if an open door inside of her had suddenly become a slivered pass-through.

"No," she would say matter-of-factly. "I just want to make sure the car gets packed up before we leave."

"Dad?" I would ask, as I watched him place his briefcase on the floor, sure there were bricks loaded inside of it. "Did something bad happen?"

"Everything is fine, Steph," he would say as I watched him walk slowly upstairs.

When they tell you how the world works, all you have to do is believe them. And when they tell you who you are, as well as what you're seeing and feeling, all you have to do is agree.

I was a Pavlovian child. Over time I learned to simply ignore the cues coming from my body, and then my body as a whole. I disconnected from my instinctual sense of the world, as well as the part of my identity that was building atop those senses. Ironically, that was the only way things made any sense. I shifted away from feeling and into the world of thinking, leaving behind the emotional in exchange for the intellectual.

All so the world could move a little quicker. All so everything was just a little bit easier. All so that things would make sense. With my mother, the fibbing came easily—it was just an extension of what I had already learned.

There was a small line at the checkout. As we waited I watched my mother examine the contents of our cart. After a few moments she looked over to me and frowned.

"This isn't ours," she said, pointing at the bottle of Baileys. "Are you sure this is ours?"

Moving slowly, enduring a thing, holding someone's hand until they understand, all while being conscious of the fact that they may never get there, is hard. Alzheimer's makes it even harder because you know "there" is a place they once couldn't imagine forgetting. To move through the truth of this disease is excruciating. As Marie Howe says, "It hurts to be present."

I wasn't trying to pull the wool over my mother's eyes, I was trying to pull the wool up and over mine. Because all of her, and all of it, was becoming so very difficult to endure. I wasn't trying to make it easier for my mother. I was trying to make it easier for myself. I was trying to move a little quicker. I didn't know yet that discomfort could be a doorway, nor did I know how quickly anger could clear a path home.

I ignored what my body was telling me—that my mother could sense when I was lying—and I told myself it would be easier for her that way. I lied. To both of us.

"You're right," I said. "It isn't ours. But I'm buying it as a gift for someone."

"Oh," she said. "That's nice. Are we meeting someone?"

I nodded and paid for our things. The bell rang again as we walked out the door.

We drove for a little less than a mile before getting back out of the car.

"Why are we stopping?" she asked.

"Because I want to take a photo," I said. "Come on. Come stand over here."

We had arrived at the Roosevelt Arch, otherwise known as the northern entrance of Yellowstone National Park.

They say the national parks belong to all of us, but there's a reason you have to have something called a visitor pass in order to enter. The park itself was established and signed into law by President Ulysses S. Grant in 1872, but for thousands of years prior to that, the land had been known by multiple Native American tribes—ancestors of the contemporary Blackfeet (Niitsítapi), Cayuse, Coeur d'Alene (Schitsu'umsh), Nez Perce (Nimiipuu), Shoshone, and Umatilla, among others. The Roosevelt Arch is located on land that was, and still is, part of the Cheyenne and Crow (Apsáalooke) nations.

From the arch, my mother and I drove through the park gates and on toward Canyon Village. We had just enough time for a hike before setting up camp, and I thought something around Yellowstone's Grand Canyon would be great. We chose the Brink of the Lower Falls Trail, a steep switchback that leads to an observation platform where you can catch the spray and the roar of the falls, as well as Red Rock Point, a mile and a half of paved trail and wooden steps that descend a bit further into the belly of the canyon.

The parking lot was jammed, as were the paths. The whole hike felt like a procession of sorts. Although the views were astounding, this didn't feel like the wilderness. It felt like a tourist attraction, like we were at an amusement park—only the bears (if we saw them) would be real, and the roller coasters would be replaced with a lineup of cars.

We caught our breath at the top of the hike and paused at the water fountains to fill our empty bottles. My mom asked me where the bathroom was and I pointed over to an area adjacent to the parking lot. There was a lengthy line of people.

"I'll wait," said my mom. "Maybe there will be a little bush somewhere."

It seemed both of us were happy to drive away from the crowds. We headed back in the direction we came, found a very quiet rest stop with a toilet, and then, about forty minutes later, we started up a steep, winding road toward our campsite. The first road led to another, which led to another, and we eventually found ourselves off pavement and on a single-lane gravel road. A few miles in, we took a slight left and ended up at a small plateau in some low, rolling hills just beyond the park. This would be home for the next few days—a breathtaking sagebrush steppe well away from the throngs.

We paid our fees and picked a flat, grassy site that smelled as if it had been dipped in pine and wild rosemary. There was a small creek just across the road that seemed to be in conversation with a series of aspen trees running along its banks—a gentle babble responded to secretive whispers. We sat down at the picnic table designated for our campsite and listened for some time. A warm wind came in from the south, shaking a dusty scent from the aspens into the air.

"What are we going to do here?" my mother asked, scanning the area.

"We're going to sleep here," I replied.

She scanned the area again.

"Here?!" she asked. "But there's no house. There's no bed."

I reminded her that we would be camping, while gesturing to the handful of other people scattered in the distance.

"Like them," I said, pointing to their tents.

"Do we have one of those?" she asked.

I nodded as I lifted the back gate of the car, reaching in to grab the tent.

"Will you help me set it up?" I asked.

She walked over to me. Her hands were held out to help, but I could tell she was concerned about how we were going to turn the nylon bag I was holding into what those people over there had.

I told her to pull the bag open and lay everything out on the ground. She did as instructed, slowly examining each item as it came out—the tent, the rain fly, the footprint, stakes, and poles. She looked toward the other campsites. She looked back to the pile of things in front of her. She looked up at me. She was still very concerned.

"Let's start with the footprint," I told her, as I pulled it from its small bag.

My mother was dazzled by what proceeded. The shaking, the laying flat, the poles that clicked into place. The sliding through, the pulling taut, the pushing in and zipping up. When the tent was erect, she stood in front of it. She was beaming. I added our sleeping pads and bags, and just to tip her over the edge of her own amazement, I showed her how we were going to make pillows out of our jackets.

She was very pleased with our handiwork. And then, after a few moments, she forgot all about it and went to go sit at the picnic table at the edge of our site.

"Is it time for bed?" she asked, looking down at her watch to see what information it had for her about what to do next.

It was just after five o'clock. The sky was still bright with the day's sun.

"Are you tired?" I asked.

"No," she said. "Not really. But what do we do now?"

"Well," I said. "We make dinner. And maybe have a drink?"

"We have drinks!" she clamored.

I walked over to the car and pulled the bottle of Baileys from the cooler.

"Here . . ." I said, handing her the bottle as I leaned in a little further, looking for the cups. "Hold this."

When I turned back a few seconds later, cups in hand, I couldn't help but laugh. There was my mother, the nondrinker, the woman who taught me table manners that, to this day, I am complimented on—and she was swigging Baileys directly from the bottle.

"Mom!" I laughed. "Do you want a cup?"

"Pffft, I don't care," she said, after lowering the bottle. "I'm cheeky, you know. Where do you think you got it all from? From me. That's where."

They say that people with various forms of dementia, including Alzheimer's, lose their filter. Apparently, this was my Baileys-loving mother without hers.

I wonder what else I might see, I thought to myself. *I wonder what else she might say.*

I brought out our stove and made us a freeze-dried backpacking meal for dinner—salmon pasta with pesto sauce. We ate in our camping chairs as we watched the sky bruise, shifting color from a bright cerulean to a golden amethyst. I rinsed and dried our dishes, popped everything back into the car, and pulled out a headlamp in preparation for sundown. When I walked back over I found my mother in the midst of a lively conversation with a mosquito.

"You land one more time and I'll slaughter you!" she warned, as the insect fed from her thigh.

I lightly slapped her leg, killing the mosquito.

"Oh," she said in relief. "Thank you. They're biting me all over."

I was suddenly filled with a flash of images: My mother hitting my tiny arms and legs as the sun went down on those summer nights near the lake. My mother's hand over my eyes. "Close your mouth," she would say as she sprayed me with insect repellent. My mother wrapping every limb of me in a large beach towel and pulling me into her lap. The lessons about how to make tiny x's over top of the bugbites by digging my fingernail into my skin. "It's better than scratching," she would say. "If you scratch it, it will itch even more. Just make an x and then leave it alone."

"Here," I said, as I knelt down in the grass beside her. "Make an x."

I pressed my fingernail into her skin, right over the bugbite.

"There's one line," I said, as I started in on the next. "And here's the other."

"Oh, that feels so good," she said.

She grabbed my hand and looked into my eyes.

"Where did you learn how to do that?" she asked.

I looked right back at her.

"My mom taught me," I said.

"Good mama," she responded. "That's a good mama."

In that moment, I wondered who she thought I was. Some familiar woman? Some kind stranger, kneeling in the grass? Some passerby who knew about mosquitos and what it was like to be raised by a good mama?

Twenty minutes later I tucked my mother into bed. She fell asleep quickly underneath a deep, indigo-colored sky. I wasn't too far behind.

When I woke the next morning, my mom was still sleeping soundly. She looked so peaceful. I crept out of the tent as quietly as possible and started in on making coffee and hard-boiled eggs in the chilly Montana air. As the water boiled, I sat back and watched the sun rise up over the mountains. I noticed the dew on the grass as it slowly turned to mist—a gentle blanket of it hovering above the ground. I sipped my first cup of coffee and watched the remnants of the night as they evaporated right before my eyes—or maybe I was watching the day producing itself. It was hard to tell. Regardless, I was glad to have seen it.

"Attention is the beginning of devotion," wrote Mary Oliver in her final collection of essays.

About thirty silent minutes passed before I heard a zipper and watched as my mother's head poked out from the flap of our bright orange tent. She looked left, examining the world in front of her, before pausing and turning her head to the right. She had a curious look on her face, one that told me she had no idea where she was. Her short hair was standing up at the back, a regular morning do for my mother, as well as a sign of a night well slept.

"Good morning, Mom," I said from my camping chair.

"Oh, hi!" she said as she spotted me. "It's you. Where are we?"

"We're in heaven, I think."

Was that a lie? I didn't think so, but I couldn't be sure.

I watched as my mother slipped on her running shoes, stood up, and looked around.

"I think so too," she replied. "I'm in my pajamas in heaven!"

I handed her a large metal mug filled with warm oatmeal and told her the plan for the day.

"We're going horseback riding," I said. "We've got to leave in about half an hour."

"Leave heaven?" she asked in earnest.

"Just temporarily," I said.

"Will I need my purse?" she asked, as she started looking around. "Where *is* my purse?"

6

A Thousand Miles of Wilderness

When we pulled into the horse corral near the northern entrance of Yellowstone we were met by our guide, David—a well-muscled peach from Georgia. David was a young Brad Pitt. David had a thick southern accent and wore fine leather chaps over the top of his pair of Wranglers. It was very quickly confirmed . . . we had not left heaven.

My mom and I were directed to a small pen where eight or so people had already gathered. David, along with the other guides on the team, took us through the safety instructions for our ride. Partway through, my mom leaned into me and flicked her eyebrows up and down. My mom also liked David.

We were set to be out riding for a number of hours. Our trip would take us well into the Yellowstone backcountry.

"And the most important thing," said David, "is to remember the name of your horse."

If we needed help while on the ride we were to say the name of our horse at high volume, so as to alert one of the guides.

"We get a fair number of y'all through here in a summer. Hard to remember all your names, so we focus on the horses."

Everyone nodded. I nodded. I looked over to my mother. She was nodding too. But I knew she wasn't taking this in. She would not remember anything from the safety talk, nor would she remember the name of her horse. As we walked from the small pen to a larger enclosure where the horses were waiting, I pulled David aside.

"David . . . um . . . can I?"

I was stumbling a bit on my words, but it wasn't because of David. It was because I didn't know exactly what to say or how to say it.

"It's . . . um—my mother has problems with her memory," I said.

No one in my family used the word "Alzheimer's" out loud. My brother once scolded me for doing so. I suppose it was too much of the truth—because you're not supposed to tell the truth. I mean, you're not supposed to lie either . . . but also, don't tell the truth. It will be easier for David.

I continued. "It's just, she won't remember any of that, and she definitely won't remember the name of her horse."

"Not to worry," said David. "I'll have you ride behind her. You're on Will and she's on Lippy. Can you remember that?"

"Yep."

"And what's her name, ma'am?"

"My mom's name is Sheila."

"Well," he said, pulling on a pair of beat-up leather gloves. "Between the two of us I think we've got it covered then, don't we."

I nodded. I loved David from Georgia.

Right before we left, I took a picture of my mother standing in front of her horse. It is one of my favorite photographs of her. She's wearing her bright red jeans and one of her thin, white cotton tops. Black sunglasses, and a white ball cap. And there's something about the way she is standing—her right hip jutting out, her left shoulder cocked up a notch, staring at the horse with a sort of coy sophistication. Her left hand, the one holding the horse's lead, is raised as if she's waiting for the horse to kiss the top of it. It's a very kittenish stance. Something I'd never seen from my mother.

When you look at that photo, you can tell, there isn't a chance she's rocking from heel to toe in that moment.

Once on our horses, we rode slowly through the corral and across the main road. From there, we dropped onto a well-worn trail that moved through the grasslands of the Yellowstone River valley. For about twenty minutes we rode in a smooth line through the undulating terrain before David held up his hand—a sign for us to stop. He gestured for us all to gather our horses as close together as possible so he could point out a few things. The first was the series of small dots lining the Grand Loop Road—cars driving one after another along the 250-plus miles of paved road in the park.

"Looks like a snake from down here, don't it?"

We nodded. We all loved David from Georgia.

"Y'all are in the one percent," he said. "Yellowstone sees about four million visitors a year, and just over one percent of them come off that road or the fifteen miles of boardwalk trails built around the main attractions."

"Wait, what?!" A voice came hurtling forward from the group of riders. A voice that belonged to me.

I'd read the brochure. There are 1,000 miles of backcountry trails in Yellowstone. Based on what David was saying, that meant 3,960,000 visitors were elbowing their way along the same fifteen miles of boardwalk. They were opting to see the wilderness from a distance as opposed to venturing into it, perhaps because observation and participation require very different things from us, especially when it comes to wild places.

"I know, ma'am," David replied. "There's a lot of beauty out here. Most people don't ever come to know it."

With that, David tipped his hat and nudged his horse forward. We all followed, but I couldn't quite get past that statistic. The idea that all we know are the views from the places we've paved over. The thought that we stick to designated asphalt paths where we are to watch for something spectacular, to wait, so that we can be entertained by life as it plays out for us, no participation required.

My thoughts turned almost immediately to my mother. How many trails was she made up of? And how many of them had I walked? Had I visited the backcountry of her mind, her wilderness? Had she been there herself? I was so hungry to see and know more of her.

And what about me? I grew up in a generation of girls who had been encouraged to take up space in the world, to run gallantly in the direction of our choice. But as we meandered through the dry grass of the river valley, I couldn't help but think something was missing, that somewhere I'd gone wrong. I *had* run gallantly in the direction of my choice. Many times over, in fact. But I wasn't sure if I'd ever taken all of myself along for the ride.

Right then, a scent drifted through the air. It was almost as if I could feel it brush by my shoulders and move gently across my face. It was something close to a smell I loved, a smell I was familiar with—rain on hot pavement, somewhere in the distance. But this was different. This smelled of the soil as well. It was petrichor—rain on warm earth, somewhere in the distance.

I lifted my face to the sky, and as the first fat droplet of water landed and slid down my cheek, I was struck with what seemed like an answer, a knowing of sorts. I had been encouraged to take up space in the world—but never inside of myself. I knew the boardwalks that ran across the surface of me, but I did not know the internal trails. I was familiar with all the ways in which I could harness my exterior power, but I was completely unfamiliar with what existed inside, the wilderness of my interior.

I had been taught to run in many directions but never to run fiercely in the direction of myself. I was always supposed to be running toward something else, toward someone else.

I looked at my mother, sitting on the horse in front of me. Her thin white shirt was getting drenched in what was now a warm torrent of rain. It only took a moment for everything to become transparent—my thoughts, her shirt as it stuck to her freckled skin, the cords of connection between us.

In that moment, a series of images spilled forth from my imagination—all of them showing me my mother on the surface of herself, cut off somehow from her internal trails. She was young—the version of her I saw in my head—eighteen or nineteen years old. Her skin was smooth. Her cheeks were full.

These images left me with a clear impression that my mother, too, had run away from herself, or at least parts of herself. That she had locked a series of internal doors. And it made sense that this would have occurred in her late teens, in 1966, in the months leading up to the birth of my eldest brother, as well as those that followed. This felt, to me, like the root of her withholding.

As I sat atop my horse I felt my hands begin to tremble. A sign, that her withholding was somehow tethered to my own.

Our succession of horses paused, and all of the riders, including myself and my mother, looked up at the sky. Sheets of rain came barreling down, and we soaked it up, we let the empty parts of ourselves fill in that valley. The whole group of us—strangers quenching a thirst we didn't know we had, feeling relief from tension we didn't know we'd been carrying. And then the storm was gone. The rain moved out as swiftly as it had moved in. Every bit of it—the clouds, the scent, every single drop—it all moved together in a singular direction. Nature was showing my mother and I what was possible.

"That'll make some goo-ood mud for them bison to roll 'round in," said David as he started back in on the trail.

We had only been riding for another few moments when I saw David's hand go up again. We paused before he motioned for us to move slowly around the bend.

"Speak of the devil," he said. "Slow and steady, ladies and gents. Slow and steady."

A herd of bison stood before us in the scrub. They were a ways off from our trail but close enough that David was suggesting some caution. We plodded forward, and as we did I stared. I could not look away from these animals. There were fifty or so spread out across the plain—some small, some large, some gargantuan. A handful were just babies, tall, gangly calves.

This seemed like a large group to me, but David reminded all of us it was small in the greater historical context.

"About five thousand live in the park today," he said. "But four, five hundred years ago there were millions. These creatures . . . they've been decimated. At the turn of the century there were only about twenty or so of 'em left in Yellowstone. You ask me, it's a devastation and a miracle all wrapped in one."

These animals were all but extinct. They were almost erased and nearly forgotten. And then, at the last minute, at the eleventh hour, something was remembered. Something moved in to protect what remained. What happened to the bison in Yellowstone, on the plains of this land, was as close to a resurrection as something can be.

I stared at the herd. I looked into their prehistoric eyes. It became immediately clear. They knew things we didn't. They know things we don't. When a living thing locks eyes with its own extinction, it learns some things in the process. The instant we came across them, I understood they were wiser than me, bigger than me.

The only way I could possibly be convinced that it was the other way around—that it was me that was bigger than them—is if I had a well inside of me, a reservoir of unspoken, unprocessed, and undealt-with anger.

It is clear upon seeing them, upon hearing them breathe, upon feeling the expanse of air that stands still as you pass them—they have carried things we haven't, they have survived the unspeakable, sacrifice runs through their blood. They don't need words to know their desire, a desire to run gallantly through a wilderness that is all their own, a fierce yearning to thunder through the backcountry. Bison will adapt, they will figure out a way to deliver themselves into freedom. They've done it before and they will do it again.

The Blackfeet have an extraordinary legend that describes how their people came to honor the bison prior to a hunt. The myth tells the origin story of a prominent ritual that is, still to this day, performed by the Blackfeet Nation as their way of showing reverence and respect for the sacrifices the bison have made. The crux of it is a dance. The Blackfeet dance for the bison. They dance in a way that brings the spirit of the bison back to life.

I want to dance for my mother. I want to dance for every day she loses. For every memory she loses, a sacrifice—on behalf of what or whom I can only fleetingly grasp.

A dear friend recently wrote a short note to me, to comfort me in the midst of losing my mother.

"Steph," she said, "isn't every day a resurrection when the one before is dead, gone forever from her mind?"

My mother is a bison. She is making a ritual offering. Her days are a devastation and miracle all wrapped in one.

I looked over to my mother as she was watching the herd—looking at them not in awe but in knowing. Some wordless language was moving between them. I felt the whispers of it on my skin.

I wanted to know what they knew and could not say. I wanted to learn this language, to translate whatever was being exchanged across the grass, across the cavernous wallows on the Yellowstone plains, between my mother and the bison. In that moment, I could have sworn it, the bison were telling her how to move from the surface of her being, so as to thunder through her very own backcountry, what sacrifices she might have to make to deliver herself once again.

After we got off our horses that day and were walking to the car, I felt an urge building inside of me. Something was telling me to keep going, to keep walking, to walk until I came upon the thousand miles of wilderness that existed in my mother. And to let that lead me to the thousand miles of wilderness that lives inside of me. I was to run gallantly in that direction. I was to dance when I arrived.

I wiped a tear from my face as I unlocked the car.

But I'm afraid, I said to whoever was out there listening. *By the time I get there, I'm afraid she'll be gone.*

I was so scared that I'd missed my chance to really know my mother, to see and understand her. I was afraid I would never have the opportunity to use that information to unlock parts of myself, to see and understand me. I was fearful that both of us would somehow be lost.

A voice came back to me by way of the wind. *She'll be gone regardless,* it replied. *At least this way there's a chance at resurrection.*

There was a mystery living inside my mother. And in that moment, I felt certain it was my job to unearth it, to venture off the pavement and discover what was living in the thousand miles of wilderness that made all of her up, from the source of her river to the valley bottom that held it.

7

All the Way Around

My mother is sitting, slightly hunched over, at the picnic table in our campsite. She's focused, immersed in the coloring book we purchased for her at the airport. The red jeans she wore on the horseback ride are slightly dirty, as is her white shirt, which has a pale green stain down the front of it—a spill from last night's dinner.

When I ask her how her day was, she looks down at her clothes, as they hold more evidence about what took place than her brain does.

"It was good," she said. "But I got a bit dirty on the bike ride."

We had not been bike riding.

"And I liked my lunch too!" she added while examining the stain on her shirt. Within a few seconds she is lost in the pages of her coloring book again.

I don't know whether my mother is moving further and further away from herself, or if she's walking back into her center. It's hard to tell with this disease. Maybe it's both. Maybe she's losing some things and finding others. Maybe this is what death looks like in slow motion. Maybe, if we stopped moving so fast, it's what aliveness really is—an infinity loop that moves us into and out of something at once. My mother is a collection of helical ribbons moving simultaneously this way and that.

I moved to the other side of the picnic table and started making dinner. Midway through I felt the wind pick up. I watched the flame on our camping stove as it trembled underneath a pot of soup. After we ate and washed everything up, the light shifted and the temperature dropped. It was sudden. I assumed a cloud or two had rolled in and was casting a shadow. But when I looked up, I didn't see a cloud or two, I saw the whole sky, ominously closing in on itself. I immediately began to load our things into the back of the car.

"Let's put the coloring away," I said to my mom. "It looks like it might rain again."

I moved everything we didn't need or didn't want wet under cover, hustled us through teeth brushing and face washing, and climbed with my mother into the tent. I showed her how to wriggle out of her clothes and into her pajamas—a repeat lesson from the night before—and then I zipped her up in her bright pink sleeping bag. It was still on the early side, but she was asleep before the first raindrop fell.

As she dozed beside me I heard thunder cracking in the distance. I peeked my head out of the tent and looked up to the sky above us. It seemed to be filling and letting go all in one moment. It was like watching an ocean in the sky—giant, Prussian-colored waves being pulled from the darkness, before cresting and crashing together. Clouds rolled up above us while thunder boomed down the mountains in the distance. The reverberations of each could be felt through the air as well as the ground underneath us.

I pulled my head back into the tent, zipped myself into my sleeping bag, and lay listening to the storm unfold, feeling both scared and relieved.

That night I had a dream. My mother and I were in a tent together. Unlike our actual tent, the one in the dream was large enough to stand in. I was lying down and my mom stood over me, very close to my feet. We were gazing softly at one another. And then, all of a sudden, she opened her mouth and started to scream. The sound poured out of her, flying from her mouth like a tumble of ropes.

Although I stayed lying down in the dream, I could feel panic tearing through my body. A panic that came with questions: Was she scared? Was she mad? Was she hurt?

No answers arrived, but after a few seconds my body flooded with relief. My mother was still screaming, but I took a deep breath and closed my eyes. As soon as they were closed, the screaming stopped, and I took another deep breath. When I reopened my eyes, still in the dream, I looked to my feet then gazed up. My mother was gone, and standing in her place was a huge black bear.

The image jolted me awake. I sat straight up in my sleeping bag, my heart racing. It was pitch black inside our tent. If an actual bear had been standing in front of me, I would not have been able to see it. I reached into the side pocket of the tent, grabbed for my phone, and pressed the home button for a bit of light.

There was no bear.

"That felt so real," I whispered to myself, as I placed my hand on my chest.

I took a deep breath and put my phone back in the tent pocket. I lay back down and waited for my heartbeat to slow. All I could hear was the sound of my mother breathing softly beside me.

How many times have I been comforted by the sound of her breath? I thought as I drifted back to sleep.

When I woke up in the morning my whole being was inundated with the memory of the dream. It felt viscerally real. For a moment, while shaking off my sleepiness, I wondered if something had actually happened in the night.

"How did you sleep?" I asked my mom, part of me thinking she might admit to having woken up in the night, or that maybe she would say, "Oh my gosh, remember the bear!"

She shrugged.

"Good, I think. I don't really know." She smiled at me. "It's so cozy in here," she added.

My mother never really had dreams, or maybe she did and just didn't remember them. I was, and still am, a vivid dreamer. I see colors and textures. I can taste and sometimes smell in a dream. They come back to me in well-detailed flashes—not unlike a stop-motion film. The remembrance rises up from some place in my body, and all of a sudden—*snap, snap, snap*—I'll have the whole dream in my mind.

"Granny dreams like that," my mother would tell me as I recounted my dreams to her as a child. And then she would add, "I don't know if I've ever remembered a dream."

I found this hard to believe. My dreams have been guideposts for my entire existence. I cannot imagine my life or my ability to make any sense of it without the movies that play inside of my head through the night.

That being said, I wasn't sure what to make of my mother's screams, nor the image I had of her becoming a bear. So I tucked the dream away for the time being, sensing that the answers would become clear over time.

My mother and I established a morning routine with ease. I would wake up almost as soon as the sun started peeking into the tent. My mom would be sound asleep. Some mornings I let her stay curled in her sleeping bag, but on most mornings I would sort of stare her awake.

"Morning, Mom!" I would whisper with excitement.

She would smile back and then make some sort of comment about her coziness. She would still be in her sleeping bag, unmoved in the night, the zipper done all the way up, and the down hood pulled up over her head. She looked like a happy seal that had been swaddled in a magenta-colored puffy.

She would look around—sleepily gathering information on where she was, and what, exactly, was happening.

"We're camping," I would remind her. "In a tent."

And then at some point she would giggle.

"Brian would hate this," she would say, referring to my father, before laughing some more. "He would absolutely hate this."

From there, I would unzip her sleeping bag for her and fill her in on the plans for the day.

"Do I wear this?" she would ask, while examining her pajamas. "I don't think I should wear this."

"I don't think so either," I would say before handing her the pile of clothes we had picked out together the night before.

Once outside, we would find a place to pee, before washing our hands and then faces. When that was done, we pulled things from the back of the car—the camping stove, the coffee, the three-gallon container of water. I would fill the pot, light the stove, and boil the water.

At some point, I would hand my mom a hard-boiled egg and tell her it was the kind you could peel. She would eat the egg while I poured some leftover water over my coffee, and the rest into the large metal camping mugs that had been filled with dried instant oats and a spoon.

"Careful," I'd say as I handed her a mug. "It's hot."

How many times had my mother laid out clothes the night before, instructed me on plans for the day, made breakfast, tested temperatures, handed me food? All of this felt as though time had somehow been folded, this moment lining up with that moment, only somehow, in the midst of it all, the roles had been reversed.

Is this why we return to our mothers? I wondered. *To take care of them as they took care of us?*

I didn't feel ready for this job. I wanted time to fold back in again. I wanted things to go back to the way they were.

After we ate, I would rinse our dishes and put all of the food back in the cooler inside of our car, tucking the camping stove and dishes beside it.

"What do we do now?" she would ask before awaiting instructions, her arms and hands relaxed at her side.

A good little girl, an obedient child. I wondered if I had been the same.

On the mornings we were driving somewhere new, I would tell my mother we had to pack up the tent.

"What tent?" she would ask, before pointing to the tent. "This thing? Pack this up?"

I would nod, a gesture that was immediately met with questions about how we might accomplish said task. Taking the tent apart was just as mystifying to my mother as setting it up.

A tent, once erect, does not look like a thing that folds very easily. She would stare at it, and I could see her trying to wrap her brain around what might come next. A huge volume of my mother's energy would move up from her body before settling densely into her furrowed brow, moving left to right, left to right in some attempt to figure it out. It was like watching someone as they tried to complete a four-piece puzzle using only two pieces.

"Before we fold it up, we have to take it apart," I would say as I began pulling up stakes and sliding out tent poles. And just before showing her how to unsnap the poles and fold them into segments, my mother would panic.

"Oh. Oh . . ." she would say. "Don't break them. That's gonna bre—"

"It won't break them, Mom. It's how they work."

I would pull and fold, pull and fold. My mother was astonished by this. These were the missing puzzle pieces.

"Look at that!" she would cry. "That's wonderful."

What followed would be my favorite part of the day.

The backbone of my family, the tent pole if you will, was consistency. Routines on repeat. Reliable patterns on which the fabric of our story and our love and our laughter could be stretched.

I could count on the fact that my dad would wash his car in the driveway each Sunday. I can see him standing at the basement sink filling a bucket with warm water and soap. I can feel the large yellow sponge in my hand on the days I was recruited to help.

I could also count on the smell of something baking—nine times out of ten, some delicious cookie dough scent would hit my nose as soon as I got to the back door of our house after school. I can hear the oven door squeaking open, the sound of cookies sliding from a tray to a cooling rack.

I have hundreds if not thousands of memories just like this, repeated experiences that have been smoothed into the grooves of my neurocircuitry. The foundation of my safety was built on top of these moments, these reliable constants that made up our everyday life. The sensation of being able to count on things has been deeply engrained. It's one of the reasons I trust the world around me. It's one of the reasons I call myself privileged—a sense of safety was sewn into my existence.

There is one image, though, that stands out from all the rest—it is of my mother as she folded the laundry. It is written in my brain in permanent ink. To me it was magic. The way she would match up and then roll a pair of socks together. The perfect squares she would make out of crumpled T-shirts. The tinier squares she would make out of boxer shorts and small pairs of underpants. Sheets, towels, pillowcases, sweatshirts. The pants, ran long, folded at the waist and then in half, smoothed over top of her legs, and folded again. A fitted sheet, turned into a flawless rectangle with even, rounded edges.

I used to watch her hands as they ran across cotton, smoothing things, fixing bumps and ridges, wiping away a flaw in the fabric with the slightest shift of her hand. And her face—it was calm and relaxed, it was meditative. I always got the sense she was doing more than the laundry, but I never knew exactly what.

She did the same with the tent. Once the poles were removed and it was just a pile of fabric on the ground, I would turn to her.

"Now we can fold it," I'd say.

She would smile, nod, and kneel down in front of the pile. The memory in her muscles knew what to do. She pulled at the edges, smoothed this bit and that, and then folded one side to meet the other. She grabbed the corners, shook it out, and laid it back down, before smoothing and folding again. She stood up, handing me two corners.

"Hold these," she would say with a clear voice—no questions, no wondering, no veil of Alzheimer's in sight.

I could hear her hands run down the fabric and I could feel

her find the bottom edge—she grabbed it gently and lifted it back up. Her hands moving toward mine.

"Give me those," she would say as I handed her my corners and watched her fold everything inward—once and then twice to a final neat square.

Her hands worked quickly, but it wasn't her hands I was watching, it was her face. There was no furrowed brow, no searching left to right in her brain. Her jawbone relaxed, her facial muscles went slack, a sense of peace washed over her. I felt like I was watching an ancient ritual.

I sat and watched as she tackled the rain fly as well as the imprint. As I sipped my coffee, lines from a Rilke poem moved through my head: *I want to unfold. Let no place in me hold itself closed.* I wondered, what parts of herself had my mother folded inward? What exactly had she tucked into the creases of T-shirts and jeans?

This had been my motto. For the previous ten years, perhaps my whole life, I had been focused on unfolding, unleashing, becoming unrestrained. There had been a giant push outward. It felt to me that my mother had done the opposite. That she had turned inward, tucked under, rolled toward the interior walls. We ourselves had moved in two different directions at once.

There were things we both did not want the world to see, parts of ourselves we wanted kept hidden. My mother held herself closed using silence. I held myself closed using noise, unending distraction. Her learned instinct was to rush in, to label it private, to not utter a word. Mine had been to rush out, to create a diversion, to fill the space with a story.

Maybe she knew of a vastness somewhere inside the internal, some space of release she could show me. And maybe I knew of stillness inside the external, a kind of comfort within the exposure that I could show her.

It wasn't hard to believe we might need both things.

Rivers need water rushing in and rushing out.

Trees need roots as well as a crown.

Igneous rock, like the obsidian found in the crown of the Yellowstone caldera, needed both hot and cold to become what it became.

And here's the thing about moving in opposite directions—if you run north for long enough, you end up in the south. And if you run south, you'll find the north at the end of the line. Somewhere along the way my mother and I were set to run into each other. Perhaps I had been returning to my mother all along. Perhaps I hadn't been riding an ebb tide, but rather taking the long route, all the way around.

Later that day, we got in the car. I instructed my mother on where to place her purse and how to buckle herself in. And together, we drove north.

8

Gossamer Wings

*Into the underland we have long placed that
which we fear and wish to lose, and that
which we love and wish to save.*

—ROBERT MACFARLANE

The questions started as soon as we pulled onto the road. We
had a four- or five-hour drive from Yellowstone to Missoula,
Montana, and about four or five hours of that time was spent
in an exhausting round-robin of questions and answers. Our
time in the car was becoming increasingly frustrating.

"Where are we going?" my mother asked as we started
our drive.

"We're headed to Missoula," I said. "It's a city in Montana."

"That's a weird sounding place," she said. "That's here?"
she added.

"Well not here, exactly, but it's where we're going."

About ten seconds later she asked the question again before moving on to a new one.

"I don't think I've been here before," she said. "Where are we?"

"Montana, Mom. We're in Montana. And you're right. You've never been here."

"Oh," she said as she looked out the window. About a minute passed. "Where ARE we?" she said, clearly perplexed.

"We're in Montana, Mom. And we're going to Missoula."

"Miss. Oula. Is that a person? Do you know her?"

"Nope."

"Are we staying with her tonight?"

"Sort of," I said with a laugh, searching for the levity in what was becoming an exasperating amount of repetition.

She paused again. "This trip is so weird."

Another minute later, she dove in again. "Where are—"

"I don't know, Mom," I said, cutting her off. "But isn't it nice?"

"It is nice. This place is very nice." She sat calmly in her seat for a few moments before asking what day it was.

"It's Tuesday," I said.

A few seconds later, she repeated the question, and I repeated my answer. "It's Tuesday, Mom. Yesterday was Monday."

"Oh."

It came a third time. "What day is it?" she asked.

"What day do you want it to be?"

She thought about that for a moment and then turned to

me. I kept my eyes on the road, hoping she would leave her questions on the flats of the I-90. She didn't.

"But what day is it?" she asked.

"It's the day we spend loving each other."

"Oh, that's a good day," she said with a giggle.

My mother was losing her mind and I was losing my patience, something my brother had warned me about, something I brushed off, thinking I would be able to handle it with ease.

A few months before the trip, I drove out to Palm Desert to visit my brother along with his wife and two kids. They were there on vacation for a week, visiting her side of the family. Upon arrival, we gathered in the kitchen and I filled my brother in on my plans, the details of where I would be taking Mom and how long we'd be gone. As I talked, my brother was futzing about—he was moving things, searching for something, filling sippy cups, and wiping fingerprints from the door of the fridge before tackling the handle.

"So that's the gist," I said, wrapping up a description of the trip. "We'll be gone for two weeks."

"Two weeks?" he asked, while he grabbed a small backpack from the floor and moved it to the countertop.

"Yeah. Just under actually."

"That's going to be hard," he said, while emptying the contents of the backpack.

"Hard why?" I asked.

He walked over to the other side of the kitchen and grabbed a glass, half-full with water, from the sink.

"You're just going to have to listen to the same questions again and again."

He poured the water out, walked over to the fridge, and filled the glass half-full with juice.

"Well, maybe that's what I need," I said.

My brother didn't respond, so I did what I do and I filled the space with more words.

"Maybe I'm supposed to have the same questions asked over and over again," I said. "Maybe that's the only way things really sink in."

My brother's futzing escalated a level. I understood this to be his final response. He handed the glass of juice to his daughter.

"Drink this," he said to her, before shouting to his wife across the room in regard to the whereabouts of the sunscreen.

He didn't move in two directions at once. He moved in one. He left the conversation, and I followed him. He was my big brother; my whole life had been about following him to various places, in various ways. It was a pattern I found hard to break free from, even in our adulthood.

As my mother and I were approaching downtown Missoula, she asked another question.

"Where are the kids?" she said, her voice laced with concern.

"What kids?" I asked, as I started looking for a good place to park. "Whose kids?"

"Your kids," she said. "Where are your kids?"

"Oh. Mom. I don't have any kids."

"Why not?" she asked pointedly.

I wasn't quite sure how to respond.

My mother asked me this question numerous times that day. And the day after. And the next one too.

"Where are your kids?" she would say.

"I don't have any kids," I would offer in response.

"You don't have kids? I thought you had kids."

"Nope. No kids."

"Why not?" she would ask, completely perplexed.

"Where are your kids?"

"We don't have any."

"But I thought they were sleeping."

"No, Mom. Those are someone else's kids."

"So, who's with your kids?"

"Mom. No. I don't have any kids."

"Oh. But you will, right? You'll have some, right?"

"I don't think so."

"Oh . . ."

Then again: "Where are your kids?"

"Mom. I don't have any kids."

"Oh no . . . why not?"

These questions came at me like a never-ending set of waves for the duration of the trip, as well as in almost every interaction we've had since. Every visit, every overnight stay, every time I spend more than ten minutes with my mother, it's, "Where are your kids?" and "Why don't you have kids?"

If there are two questions a childless woman in her thirties does not want to be asked and does not want to answer, it is those two questions. In the last four years, my mother has asked them hundreds of times. Over and over and over.

The truth is, I wasn't getting tired of my mother's repetitive questions. I was getting tired of the ones that made me question myself.

I spotted what looked like a small wine bar on the other side of the street, and I parked the car. I turned to my mom and told her, rather sharply, that it was time for lunch. She nodded.

Once we were out of the car, I grabbed her hand, checked for traffic, and when it was all clear, I pulled us swiftly across the street. I needed a glass of wine, something that would keep my frustration from tipping over into anger.

We settled in at a table by the window and I ordered us each a drink—a large pour for me, a margarita, no salt, for her—as well as a handful of things to share for lunch.

My mother placed her hands gently in her lap and sat across from me silently. She had picked up on my frustration. When our drinks came, she slurped hers back with gusto and asked if she could have another.

"Of course, you can," I said, as I slowly sipped my wine.

Our server brought my mother's second drink. This time it came with a miniature, paper umbrella, which my mother promptly plucked out of the glass.

"What is this?" she asked.

"It's an umbrella," I said.

"But it's not raining," she said, while she slid it open and closed. "And this . . . this looks like it would fall apart if it got wet."

I laughed. It's ridiculous really—an umbrella for a drink.

"It must be for pretend," she added. "Like for a dolly or something."

She placed the umbrella on the table and lifted her drink in the air.

"Cheers!" she said, with a smile. "This is so nice."

I clinked her glass and took another sip of my wine.

"I mean . . ." she continued. "This is so special. I ju—"

There was a crack in my mother's voice. I looked up and saw she was crying. Smiling, and crying.

"Mom?" I asked. "Are you okay?"

"I . . ." She paused. "I haven't felt like this in a long time," she said.

Her voice was quite different all of a sudden. Although the cracks were still there, there was no confusion. No layer of worry, or wondering. This happened on occasion—on a good day. Every once in a while, my mother came through in some unaffected version of herself. It was almost as if Alzheimer's was a jacket, and in a moment here or there, she could simply remove that jacket and place it gently on the back of her chair. This was one of those moments.

I stared into her eyes and felt my shoulders release. I hadn't realized how much tension I'd been carrying. I had forgotten that just underneath the relative stranger across from me was a woman I knew well. A woman I loved.

Mom, I thought to myself, as I watched her sitting there smiling.

"I'm having so much fun," she said, as she wiped away her tears. "I look at myself in the mirror and I don't even know who it is. This is just so special. I have to thank you."

"It is special," I said with a happy sigh, feeling awful about my earlier frustration.

"You know," she said. "I love your father—I always have—but he would never do this . . . a trip like this."

I chuckled, fully aware of just how accurate a statement that was.

"We've been on lots of adventures," she said. "But he doesn't . . . he wouldn't want to get—"

I knew my mother was searching for a word, and I knew exactly what that word was.

"DIRTY!" I said.

"YES! Dirty! He hates getting all mussied up."

She raised her hand in the air for a high five and waited until I hit her palm with mine.

I sat back, hoping there was more. Longing for a few more minutes of my mother, thirsty for her, thirsty for her words.

"Your father has been the greatest gift of my life," she continued. "He always had ideas and plans to travel here and there, and I happily went along with them. And we've had so much fun. It's just . . ." She paused for a moment. "It never occurred to me to ask Brian to do something like this."

It never occurred to her? I wondered to myself.

I felt something inside of me screech to a halt.

It never occurred to her?

My mind leapt back in time—flashing to a conversation I'd had with my dad a year or so prior.

We were talking about the first book I'd written, about the ferocity with which I chased the masculine ideal, about how hard I had tried to become "one of the guys." The conversation bled into my thoughts on modern-day feminism, the shifts that had occurred inside of myself as well as in the ideological and societal tides.

"You know," said my dad, from his corner of the couch. "Looking back, I think we treated you differently."

"What do you mean?" I asked, suddenly confused. "Treated *who* differently?"

"It wasn't a conscious thing," he said, continuing on as if he hadn't heard me. "But we treated your brothers differently than you and your sister."

My insides felt as though they had been suddenly squeezed. There was a twisting inside my stomach and then a great flare, a quivering, like an eclipse of moths had just been released inside me. They were fluttering wildly. They rose from that twisting place. They rose toward a flame—bright-colored rage in my chest. My body was not used to this feeling.

I promptly moved in two different directions at once. Inwardly, I felt chaos. Outwardly, I remained calm. I did so because I had questions, questions that I wanted answered.

"How so?" I asked quietly, a casual tone concealing my indignation.

My father continued.

"We pushed the boys," he said. "We challenged them."

The rage grew brighter. There were more moths. It was a frenzy. My insides were fleeting light and fluttering darkness.

I nodded. I was hoping there would be more, and at the very same time, I was wishing that was the end of it.

Do I want all of the truth, I thought to myself, *or just some of the truth? How much truth is too much in this instance?*

"It's just . . ." he continued. "You and your sister were both—"

He pursed his lips ever so slightly before taking a large mouthful of wine. I sat waiting as the moths ate any of the light remaining inside of me.

"You were both pretty," he said. "You were charming and good-natured. We just figured you'd both find really nice guys."

I felt them as they took over my body. I was drowning in a thousand pairs of gossamer wings.

Sitting in front of my mother, watching her sip her margarita, my thoughts flitted back to the words of my therapist: "You think you're bigger than your mother."

Doesn't everyone? a voice responded in my head. *Don't we all think we're bigger than our mothers? Isn't that what we've been taught?*

My parents thought I was pretty, charming, and good-natured.

My parents thought my contribution to this place, to this world around me, was my appearance, my ability to delight.

Their highest hope was that I turn out to be good-natured and unselfish, that I offer kindhearted support to some— did he say "nice guy"? That's what he said, right? He said I would find a nice guy.

The challenge they offered was for me to find someone who would, if I was lucky, maybe find me? Did anyone know where I was? Was anyone looking? Did anyone realize that the women were in boats somewhere, keeling this way and that in the sea?

Another memory surfaced, something more recent in time—my mother and I driving through Vancouver in the handful of months prior to this trip.

About a block away from the house, she turned to me.

"Are the boys together?" she asked.

"Yep," I said, not entirely sure what boys she was referring to but also not wanting to create confusion.

"Oh good," she said. "Let the boys play."

I paused. Something inside of me grew curious.

"What do the girls do?" I asked. "You know . . . while the boys play?"

"Oh," said my mom with a shrug. "I dunno."

She was utterly stumped by the question. And her tone was clear. It was almost as if she had added, "Why would that even matter."

My parents thought boys were bigger than girls. My parents thought a father was bigger than a mother. Nothing else mattered so long as the boys were onshore. And the women, they swallowed their rage. These were the unspoken truths— the things I'd known but never once given a name to. Looking back, I could see these truths made up the stitching of my every action.

I was handed the idea that my fulfillment, my eventual wholeness, was dependent on finding a nice guy.

Once you find him, you'll be whole.

I had anger about this, but instead of feeling it, I'd buried it. I stuffed it somewhere inside of me and attempted to make myself bigger. Looking back, I saw this everywhere—threads of it were sewn through every decision I had ever made.

The flicking away of some unnamed essence, my fierce rejection of the feminine, and the subsequent shooting down of my mother. The scaffolding, the very large pedestal I built for my father. My attempt to, as Toko-pa Turner has said, "become as Athena was, aligned with her father in order to thrive."

Once you become him, you'll be whole.

Somewhere in the bones of my parents, and their parents before them, and theirs before them, someone implanted the following proposition: the masculine > the feminine.

One was bigger than the other. My mistake was that I had believed them.

The share plates I had ordered arrived at the table. A side of fried cauliflower, a beet and burrata salad, and some roast chicken with greens.

"What is this?" my mom asked, while pointing at the cauliflower.

"That's cauliflower, Mom," I said. "Careful, it might be a bit hot."

"That's cauliflower!" she cried. "This is amazing. I would never think to make cauliflower like that."

"Right?" I agreed, noticing that somewhere along the way my mother had slipped back into her Alzheimer's jacket.

"You know," she said, "I just did what my mom did. She . . ."

My mother was searching for words. I filled them in for her.

"She steamed it," I said. "Your mother steamed the cauliflower."

"Yes! She steamed it," she said. "But how did you know that?"

"Because that's what you did. And that's what you taught me to do."

"Well," she said, matter-of-factly. "We should do it differently now. We need to do it differently."

"We sure do," I said, as I finished my glass of wine.

I've thought about becoming a mother many times, but there has always existed a small but powerful voice inside of me that has rejected the idea, each and every time it has surfaced. I have chosen to listen to that voice, not entirely knowing whose it was or where, exactly, it came from. After lunch with my mother that day, I came to understand that the voice had always been hers.

Somewhere in this life she had given me a greater than / less than comparison when it came to gender. But it wasn't that simple. In some other place or in some other way she had always been whispering to me about alternate routes, other paths, a different way to cook cauliflower. In one world she handed me a mathematical problem. In another world she handed me the proof.

It's a very confusing thing to feel as though my mother helped me build those confines and was, at the very same time, encouraging me to break them. But maybe it wasn't confusing; maybe it was the bridge her generation was destined to build. What an impossible job that would have been—working so hard to uphold the image their mothers had shown them and at the same time stretching their arms clear across some divide, trying to deliver us into a world they could not yet see.

And what a thing it must have been for her to live inside such a deep crevasse. The generation prior pushing in from one side, telling her that the very definition of love is suppression, that she mustn't burden people with her pain, all while feeling me squeezing hard from the other side, desperate for a radically different definition of love, one based on expression, on our capacity to sit with and tell all of the truth.

How big of a leap can we expect from one generation to the next? When will we begin to see our mothers based on the soil they grew up in as opposed to the patch of earth we find ourselves currently planted in? When will we understand that the divides they were reaching across were all the parts of themselves they had been denied access to?

I hadn't thought of my mother as a woman who broke outside of the confines that shaped her, but in truth she had shattered them all. They were just different confines than the ones I grew up in.

As we got back in the car, I thought of my mother and her five children—myself and the three siblings I grew up with, as well as the brother born earlier, the one we met along the way. The past, and her present and her future, pulling, pulling, pulling—a river both brought to life and stretched thin, water made to move in multiple directions at once.

And as we drove out of Missoula, I thought of the city itself. The way it sits at the convergence of five mountain ranges: the Bitterroots, the Sapphire Range, the Garnet Range, the Rattlesnake Mountains, and the Reservation Divide. Five towering ranges running toward a lake-bottom valley that no longer has any water left in it.

Not many people know that the mother of Athena was Oceanid, a woman who held the wisdom of water, both salty and sweet. She is often overlooked, so much so that in places, it appears the water has run dry. But that doesn't mean it's not there; all you have to do is look beneath the surface. A descent into the underground will often reveal a wellspring, where an unseen source, a mother lode of wisdom, has been flowing for centuries.

9

The Great Divide

My mother was sound asleep. A bear was hovering just over her body; it was about to pounce, to devour her whole. I lunged forward to get in between them, and in that very moment I realized the bear was me.

My own gasping woke me from the dream. I turned quickly, searching for my mom in the darkness of the tent. Part of me expecting her to be awake, in a panic, and possibly hurt in some way. She was none of those things.

I could hear her beside me. She was breathing gently in and out.

I wiggled my toes at the bottom of my sleeping bag, attempting to shake off the dream.

My dreams don't usually wake me, I thought before rolling to my other side and drifting back to sleep.

The dream resurfaced the next morning as a set of disoriented images and emotions. All of which I brushed aside rather quickly, as I had a big day planned, a day that required I get us ready a little earlier than normal.

About an hour or so after getting in the car, we pulled into a small gravel parking lot. The day prior, I had called a local white water rafting company to inquire about fun but gentle trips on the river.

"The Clark Fork. Alberton Gorge," said the guy on the phone. "You'll love that trip. Water's running fast on that one."

"And it's gentle?" I reiterated.

"Super gentle," he replied.

The Clark Fork is the largest river by volume in Montana. It is responsible for draining a massive region of the Rocky Mountains, allowing snow and ice and metric tons of water to flow into the mighty Columbia, and from there into the salty Pacific. It is a major artery of the west, a bloodline that surges through the land, breathing life into the surrounding basin and beyond.

The highest point in the Clark Fork's watershed runs along the Continental Divide—a geographic and hydrologic feature that has always amazed me. Snowfall and rain that land on the west of the divide melts and rushes through steep watersheds toward the Pacific Ocean. Water that lands on the east of the divide makes its way into the Missouri River, before spilling into tributaries that curl toward the ocean on the east, the Atlantic.

And it makes sense that there is a natural divide, paths that move water this way and that, but I've always been curious about the water that lands right on top. How does it decide which way to go? What elements are involved in its watershed moment? I want to know what water looks like when it surrenders. But perhaps that's the nature of it, perhaps surrender is the only way of being water knows, perhaps that's the only way it breaks.

The parking lot was empty when we arrived, and even though I saw a river to our left, I wasn't sure if we were in the right place. There were no buildings, no other cars, and I couldn't see any people.

"Are we stopping here?" asked my mom.

"I think so," I said. "Let's look around."

I got out of the car and felt the crisp air hit my face. I immediately wondered if this was a mistake. If I thought it was cold, my mom would think it wa—

"Oooh," she said, as she stepped out of the car. "It's freezing out here!"

"Let's get you zipped up," I said, as I reached for the zipper on her coat.

"What are we doing here?" she asked, her voice suggesting she would much rather be back in the warmth of the car.

"We're here to go rafting," I said, looking down a small frontage road to our right.

"Here," I added, pulling a dark grey beanie down over her head. "Follow me."

I grabbed my mother's hand and started walking down the road. As we turned the corner, I spotted what looked like two double-wides. There was a wooden deck built around them, and a sign that said MONTANA RIVER GUIDES was hung on the side.

"Looks like we're here," I announced.

I was nervous about taking my mom on this adventure. It felt like there was a lot more that could go wrong on the water than on horseback, but I reminded myself I had asked for something gentle.

"We'll be fine," I whispered to myself in reassurance, as I stepped into what looked like a makeshift tourist shop with a small check-in area. "We'll be fine."

There were two other people inside, both of whom were wearing branded apparel. One was standing behind a small countertop filling a display rack with lip balms and neoprene neck straps. The other was across the room, organizing a stack of T-shirts and hats.

"Hi, there," I said. "Is this where the Alberton trip runs out of?"

The woman behind the counter looked up.

"Oh," she said. "Sorry about that. Didn't see ya there!"

Just then another staffer walked in the door. He was wearing a plaid shirt, turquoise shorts with wet-suit leggings poking out from underneath, and a pair of worn flip-flops. He was massive. At least six foot five. Maybe taller.

"I'm Quinn," he announced. "Y'all coming on the Fork with us this morning?"

I looked up at Quinn.

"You must be my mother-daughter duo," he said.

I nodded.

"Yep, that's us," I said, as I swung my arm around my mom. "I'm Steph, and this is my mom, Sheila."

My mom scaled Quinn with her eyes.

"You're so tall," she said. "What did you eat to get that tall?"

Her question was an earnest one.

Quinn laughed, and then pointed us toward the changing rooms.

"Let's get you two suited up," he said.

Once in the stall, I helped my mom out of her clothes and into the provided wet suit and booties. Between the wiggling, pulling, yanking, and adjusting, my mother asked a lot of questions—questions about how that man got so tall, about why we were wearing these outfits, and about where she should put her purse.

I did my best to answer them all before donning my wet suit. And then, when I finally had us both sorted out, I turned back to my mother. She was standing beside me, examining what she was wearing. She was apprehensive about this look.

"Where are we going in these outfits?" she asked, as I walked her out of the changing area. "We look so weird. Are these even shoes?"

I looked at her and laughed. She was wearing a black-and-grey full-length wet suit, complete with small, split-toe booties, and a blue life jacket. A bright yellow helmet was popped over top of the grey beanie I had told her to wear earlier that morning, and she was holding on to her purse.

"I don't think you'll need that," I said, referring to the beanie. I reached over, undid her helmet, and pulled the beanie off her head. "And we can put your purse in the locker," I added. "You won't need it in the water."

"In the water?" she asked in confusion. She looked around for a while and then spotted the river down below us.

"In there?!" she shrieked, pointing toward it. "But that looks so cold!"

Quinn came walking up behind us.

"Well, Sheila," he said, as we turned to face him. "I'm hopeful we won't actually go in the water, but we will be going in some boats."

"You might get a little wet," I added. "Like a splash here or there."

I dashed back into the changing rooms, locked my mother's purse up with the rest of our things, and popped back outside. There were now three other people standing with Quinn and my mother. Our rafting group was complete.

"Looks like we're all here," he said, before gesturing to the wooden deck. "Let's gather up for a safety talk."

I put my hand on the back of my mom's arm and moved us to some benches that had a dappling of sunlight on them. I wanted to keep her as warm as possible before hitting the water.

Quinn and another guide took us through a fairly long set of safety instructions, almost all of which had me imagining my mother rag-dolling into the rapids. Apparently my mother was imagining something similar, because about halfway through the talk she leaned into me with wide eyes.

"This is a lot of things to remember," she whispered.

"Don't worry, Mom, I'll remember for you."

"You will? You can remember all that?"

"I sure hope so," I whispered back.

At the end of the talk I pulled Quinn to the side.

"Quinn," I said. "My mom—"

I swallowed hard before continuing.

"Quinn . . . my mom has Alzheimer's."

It was the first time I had said it out loud.

Quinn nodded. His eyes softened ever so slightly.

"She won't remember a thing you just said," I added. "All that self-rescue stuff—that'll be gone. This is an easy trip, right?"

Sensing my nerves, Quinn put his giant hand on my shoulder.

"Not to worry," he said. "Can she paddle?"

"You mean in the water?" I asked.

Inside my head there was a voice. *Oh god,* it said. *He thinks we might go in the water.*

"I mean, she can swim—she's never been that strong of a swimmer though."

"No," said Quinn. "I mean, can she *use* a paddle?"

"Oh!" I said, laughing. "Yes. She can paddle. She's really good with in-the-moment instructions, and she's surprisingly strong."

"Great," he said. "I'll put her on my right so she can hear me."

A handful of minutes later, I watched as the second guide helped my mom get into the bright yellow raft.

My mom repeated every instruction. She couldn't fully articulate what she was feeling, but I could tell she was as nervous as I was.

"Hold on here?" she asked, after the guide told her what to hold on to.

"Yes," said the guide. "Exactly. Hold that there."

"Sit here?" my mother asked with trepidation.

"Yes, Sheila. Right there. And then wedge your feet in between those tubes."

"Put my feet between these?" she asked.

"Yep. In between there."

"Ooh, that pinches a little," she said. "Okay. What else?"

"That's it. All you have to do is stay there."

"Stay here?" she asked in confirmation. "Okay, I'll stay right here."

I was next into the boat. They sat me directly across from my mother. Right after I held on here and wedged my feet there, I looked over to her. We were both holding our breath, taking in the smallest sips of air. And then we were each handed a small blue-and-yellow paddle.

"Hold this?" my mother asked. "Like this?"

"Just like that, Sheila," said Quinn, as he began pushing the boat off the shore. "Off we go," he announced, before hopping in himself.

My mom sat holding the paddle across her lap.

"The beautiful thing about rivers," said Quinn, "is that they take us from one place to another."

Quinn sat just behind my mother and me, in an elevated seat in the middle of the boat. He settled in quickly, reached for the large oars on either side of him, and smiled a broad smile as he looked downriver.

"You all ready for the Clark?" he asked the group, while

maneuvering the boat into the flow of the water. "She's calm here, but she's runnin' a bit wild in the gorge today!"

I looked back at Quinn. I did not want wild. I could handle wild, but my mother could not. And I could not handle my mother not handling wild.

Quinn must have seen the panic flash through my eyes.

"Don't worry," he whispered. "She can handle what comes. Always has, am I right?"

In that moment, I wasn't sure if Quinn was referring to the river, the boat, or my mother. Perhaps he was talking about all of them.

I glanced over to the other side of the boat. My mom was now staring downriver, into the gentle blue-and-green curls of the water. Her nervousness had evaporated. She was mesmerized. Water has always done that to her. She's never been an outwardly frenzied woman despite her constant worry, but something happens when she's close to the water. Her undercurrent shifts. The steady hum of worry that runs in her background subtly subsides. I feel her energy, her whole self, melt into a more fluid and natural calm. Whenever she looks out over the ocean, or at a rippling lake, or a large, rushing river—it's like a missing piece of her comes home, some unnamable part of herself sort of slips back into place. I've never fully understood it, but I've seen it happen many times—those moments where pure fluidity exists inside of my mother.

She smiled, and I took a deep breath. This is why I booked the rafting trip—the look on my mother's face when she watches the water. It makes me feel as though I can see all of her, all the way through to the stones at the bottom, to the sediment that makes up the bed underneath her.

"Mom?" I asked quietly. "Are you excited?"

She looked over to me.

"Yes," she said. Her answer had such clarity, such certainty.

"What are you excited about?" I asked.

"Whatever this is," she said, before looking back to the water.

My mother's ability to surrender astounds me. And even though we've never uttered a word between us about it, I know it comes from the way in which she first entered motherhood, a place I've always thought of as some kind of wilderness. Regardless of the route in which you enter, I can only imagine it must feel as though you're just tossed right in, like you're thrown directly into the thick of it. That you must, as you have to on a river, understand the dance between surrender and control, the grace that is involved in going with the flow of something that has a heartbeat wholly separate from your own.

My mother's route in was an interesting one. As I understand it, she was told where to sit, but I don't think she was ever handed a paddle.

My eldest brother was born on July 27, 1966. Although it happened in a hospital somewhere near Vancouver, Canada, part of me thinks it may have occurred on top of the Great Divide. My mother tumbling from that place to the salty shores of the west, my eldest brother taking a long and winding route through the plains before landing in a faraway spot just below the Great Lakes.

My parents were eighteen and nineteen years old. It was the '60s. The water rose and broke quickly. In the end, or perhaps it was the beginning, my mother chose to surrender. In many ways, she had to.

She moved in two different directions at once—it was my mother's great divide. She went west, eventually making her way back to my father. And their firstborn, a baby boy, went east by route of adoption. I can only assume that in the midst of it all, something inside of her closed—a doorway, perhaps, to her thousand miles of wilderness.

Maybe that's when she started looking at water that way, gazing wistfully, searching hopefully—for her firstborn child, as well as all the pieces of herself that must have gone missing in the process.

Once I find him, I'll be whole.

The water was moving swiftly now. Quinn was giving instructions on when to paddle and precisely how hard, and my mother was focused. She thrived when given a job to do, especially a physical one.

The boat bounced up and down between sections of frothy white water, slowing to a soft glide as we moved through deep green pools and calm eddies. Back and forth, back and forth, back and forth, until we dropped down into a deep gorge—the throat of the river. A steep canyon of grey stone and purple cliffs rose up on either side of the river, and pine trees stood tall on the ridgelines. We were in big water now, tumbling through sections of boiling water and small, rocky falls. I could hear my mother on the other side of the boat. She was shrieking in joy.

As the rapids began to slow, I heard Quinn's voice.

"You're right," he yelled from behind me. "She can paddle!"

"Look right!" he added, speaking now to the whole group.

A family of deer was scrambling through some rocky scree. As we paused in some gentler water to watch, I heard the sound of an eagle chattering somewhere up above us.

I looked over to my mom, wondering if she too had seen the deer or heard the eagle. She hadn't. With her right hand, she was holding the perimeter line of the boat. And as the rest of us were looking up, my mother's eyes were cast down. She was watching the river.

As Annie Dillard wrote, "Live water heals memories."

Later that afternoon, we drove from the outskirts of Missoula toward Kalispell and, eventually, Columbia Falls. We crossed over the Flathead River—the largest tributary of the Clark Fork—and a handful of miles later I pulled off the main highway and down a road toward the Hungry Horse Dam. I parked the car in a small lot beside a visitor's center and reached into a bag in the back seat of the car.

"Want an apple?" I asked my mom.

She nodded.

"With some cheese?" I added.

She nodded again.

"Mmmmm," she said, as she ate her snack in the front seat of the car. "Yummy in my tummy."

Once we were finished, we walked into the visitor's center. My mom looked out the viewing window while I glanced over the infographics posted on the wall. I read about how the dam's bell-mouth spillway is the largest in the world, and about how many billions of kilowatts of power the dam produces annually. And then I joined my mother at the window—the two of us staring out at the vast expanse of concrete built up before us.

We got back in the car and headed northeast. We drove through winding mountain roads—two or three hours of switchbacks. The curves were so tight you couldn't see anything around the bend until you arrived there. Back and forth, back and forth, back and forth, until we were up and over the Continental Divide.

I thought about the dam the whole time. I understood why it was built. I read about what it created and what it produced. But the visitor's center didn't have any information about what happens when the course of a river is altered in that way, when something wild is forced into some kind of shape. When part of it is told to move this way and part if it is told to move that way.

Did they forget about that? Did they forget about the power of the actual river?

We think steel and iron are sturdier than silt and clay and soil. We think concrete is stronger than water. We think if we close something off, we'll have control of everything that exists, locked behind the door. This creates a grand illusion. To those around us, we begin to look smaller than we are; we look like a stream, just a warm and trickling brook. Oh, the illusion is a strong one.

That whole morning I had been worried that my mother couldn't handle the rapids, when the truth of it was, she was the rapids. My mother was the water—the river as well as the raft. She had moved each and every one of us—myself, my father, and each of my siblings—from one place to the next.

My mother had delivered us all. She was bigger than every single one of us.

But who is going to deliver my mother? I wondered. *Who is going to carry her from one place to the next? From this life, to an ever after?*

I wasn't sure I knew anyone big enough for this job.

"Look," my mom said, while pointing out the window of the car. "There's whipping cream on those mountains."

"That's snow on the mountains, Mom."

"Who says?" she asked quickly. "I think it's whipping cream for the animals."

"You know what, Mom?" I said. "Maybe you're right."

10

Pencil Shavings and Juniper Berries

As we come to understand the symmetry
between the outer landscape and the inner
wilderness, we can't help but grieve the ways
in which our own nature has been tampered
with, denigrated, broken into obedience, and
in many cases eradicated from memory.

—TOKO-PA TURNER

It was early June. A colossal amount of snow had fallen the winter prior. The infamous but often dangerous Going-to-the-Sun Road that snakes through Glacier National Park was still covered in snow. My mother and I had no choice but to go the long way round. Although this seemed fitting given what I was learning about our dance, the consistency in my leaving as well as my lengthy return.

We were about ten miles south of the park's eastern entrance when I felt something shift—the energy, the landscape, everything. My mom did too.

"Where are we?" she asked. "Are we somewhere different?"

"No," I said, as I looked out the window, slowing the car ever so slightly. "And also yes."

I saw a handful of charred trees in the forest around us, and as we drove there were more and more. About a mile or so later, they were all charred—there wasn't so much a forest around us as rolling fields of compact dirt and ash, thin black poles, thousands of them standing there like cracked and lonely ghosts. No branches, no ability to reach out to one another, no longer a collective of evergreen anything. The whole scene was eerie.

Were these lodgepole? I thought to myself. *Or Doug fir?*

The scarring that ran across their bodies and all the way up to the tips of their crowns made it impossible to tell.

The Red Eagle burn erupted in July of 2006. It burned 34,000 acres over the summer and fall. After raging for nearly six months, it was called dead out that winter.

It's so easy for us humans to disguise our hurt, to mask our trauma, to have it appear as though nothing has happened to us. Nature is different that way. It doesn't have much of a choice in the matter. It must show us who it is in the face of its pain. It must stand in the ashes of the parts that were burned. It must grow from that place, visible sinews of past anger turned into growth and expansion.

In late 2015, someone gave my mom an adult coloring book. The book, like all adult coloring books, contained hundreds of pages of elaborately drawn scenes—gardens and forests and underwater worlds that my mom was supposed to bring to life. It was something to keep her busy. Something she could do while sitting at the kitchen table. Something she didn't have to talk to or remember the history of. It was the perfect gift.

My mother dove into coloring like I dive into the bulk candy section at the grocery store—with shocking excitement and focus. Hour after hour, day after day. My mother devoured the octopus's garden, and after that the sleepy hollow, and after that the English flower bed. She was consumed. She got completely lost. Or maybe she was getting completely found. It was hard to tell.

Within a few weeks, more books were purchased, pencil crayons were pulled out of old drawers and beat-up cases, and a slightly rusted sharpener was put back into rotation. Her sisters organized a group coloring party at Christmas that year. All four of them went to my aunt Daphne's house, coloring books in tow. There's a picture of them sitting at the dining room table really givin' 'er with their pencil crayons—my uncle Doug off to the side, holding a tray of gin martinis for the artists. If you looked at that picture, I swear you'd smell it— pencil shavings with a hint of juniper berry.

For a lengthy period of time, whenever I went home to visit my parents, I could count on the fact that my mom would be parked at the kitchen table, getting between the lines like a madwoman, like a woman who has (no pun intended) lost her mind. The assortment of green pencil crayons ground down to nubs.

"There are so many leaves," she would say while glancing at the pile of moss-colored pencil crayons, lying dead on the table.

"You don't have to color all the leaves green," I would tell her. "They can be red and brown, or yellow and orange. You just have to pretend it's fall." It would occur to me that these were likely the very things she said to me when I was little.

You just have to pretend.

"Well, that wouldn't look very good," she would say flatly, her tone suggesting I was sitting somewhere between absolutely absurd and utterly ridiculous.

Another hour or two would go by and she would place her pencil crayons on the table.

"Look," she would say, holding her right hand out for me to see. "It hurts."

My mother's right thumb and pointer finger would have deep indentations in them. Turns out that four or five or six hours straight of pushing down on a pencil crayon will leave an actual impression. It would make me wish I could do the same with her brain.

I would take her hand in mine and massage her two fingers.

"Ow, ow, ow," she would say before looking down at the page again and smiling. "Just a little bit more."

She was obsessed. An entire bag of completed coloring books sits underneath her desk in the kitchen. There's got to be a dozen or two in the stack—pages and pages she's plowed through in some prolific artistic streak. The funniest thing about it is that up until she got that first book, I had never seen my mother color. Or paint. Or draw. Not once.

Although both of her parents had substantial artistic tendencies, I'd always thought of my mother as more of an athlete than an artist. So I figured the coloring had to do with relief. Relief in finding an activity that had nothing to do with her ability to remember words, or places, or faces. Basically, I thought she was just meditating for hours at a time, coloring, because it felt good. Not once did I think it was a coping mechanism, or that the obsession was anything other than a healthy new habit. Not once, until I had a conversation with my auntie Brenda as we wandered through Glacier National Park.

I'd told my aunt Brenda about the trip as soon as I'd decided on the basic plan. She lived in Calgary at the time, just a few hours from the eastern entrance of Glacier, so I called her, wondering if she wanted to join us for a handful of days. I got an immediate yes.

We kept the whole thing a secret, which, because of Alzheimer's, was not rocket science. But we did it regardless. Both my aunt and I wanted to do something special for my mom. And for us. We wanted the whole thing to feel special.

A handful of months later there we were. My aunt was waiting for us at the campsite, having arrived early to fill the park ranger in on the secret. And lemme tell ya, as soon as my mother and I walked into the visitor's center, this park ranger was there at the ready. I gave her the name of our reservation, and when I did she got all "shaking Chihuahua" excited. Turns out she wanted something special too.

"Why is that lady being strange?" my mom whispered to me in the waiting area.

"Well, Mom, I have a surprise for you at the campsite, and this lady here knows what it is."

"You do-oooo?!" she exclaimed to both of us. "You have a surprise?!"

"I sure do," I said.

The shaking Chihuahua nodded her head. She could barely look at my mother. It felt to me like she was scared she might just blurt the whole thing out if they made eye contact. So instead she shook. In my direction.

We got back into our car and my mom couldn't help herself. She was so excited.

"For me!" she exclaimed. "You have a surprise for *me*?"

She paused to think for a moment.

"Are our husbands coming?!" she asked.

"Nope," I said. "But that's a good guess!"

From there she was stumped. She sat back, looked out the window, and within a few seconds the whole concept of the surprise was gone.

I drove us down a dirt road that ran adjacent to a small river. And then, at a campsite around the bend, I spotted my aunt's car. I slowly pulled our car into the parking spot beside hers.

"I think this is someone else's," said my mom.

"Nope. This is ours," I said. "I have a surprise for you."

"You do-oooo?!" she asked with astonishment. "Is someone else here? Is it our husbands?!"

"Nope. Not our husbands," I repeated. "You'll see . . . it's someone you know."

By this point, Brenda had spotted us and was walking toward the car.

"That person?" my mom asked, peering out the window, trying to get a better look. "Is it that person?"

"Yep. That person."

And then my mother saw her—like *saw her,* saw her.

"I know her!" she cried.

What a thing it must be to recognize something whilst living in a world of unrecognizable things.

My mother could not get out of the car fast enough. Tears were streaming down her face. She was frantic with her seat belt. As soon as the clip released, she jumped out of the car and ran, with open arms, toward her sister.

"How di . . . how did you know we would be here?" said my mom, choking back tears. "How on earth did you know we were here?"

"Steph and I planned it," said Brenda. "I drove down from Calgary last night. And LOOK . . . I've got my tent all set up over here!"

Brenda's energy has always been sparkly to me, effervescent in nature. Almost all of my memories of her include giggling. And even the memories that don't, the ones that are painful and hard, include me watching her as she reached for laughter. It's part of the reason I invited her. It's pretty easy to wade through the quicksand of Alzheimer's without laughter, without levity of any kind. In this type of quagmire, you think patience is the only weapon you're going to need, but it's not. If patience is the shield, laughter is the sword you holster to your thigh. And if anyone I knew had experience with this particular type of thigh holster, it was Brenda. She'd used it in multiple battles.

I wanted Brenda with us because of this, but I also wanted her to tell me everything she knew. Brenda would have been twelve years old in the winter of 1965 when my mom first got pregnant, and thirteen the following summer. She is one of the few people on the planet who knew my parents before, during, and after that year, and one of two people still alive who actually lived with my mom during that time.

Brenda would have borne witness to my mom and her first pregnancy. She would have seen at least one side of the story my mother had been carrying inside of her.

Brenda saw my mother as she scrambled to the top of the divide, and Brenda saw her as she came tumbling back down.

I wanted my aunt to join us in Glacier because I wanted her memories. She was the only person who could give an eyewitness account. Mom was never able to.

She had taken a black pencil crayon to that period of time. She colored over it. She blacked it out. She had redacted that whole story from her whole story.

I didn't know what Brenda knew, but I knew it had to be something, and I knew it was more than I knew. So I asked. We went on a hike the next day and I asked.

It was a cloudy morning, and the threat of rain hung low in the sky, so we opted for a meandering walk not far from our campsite. We threw our rain jackets on, filled a backpack with a few extra layers and snacks, and set out on a trail-cum-dirt road that wound its way through a handful of open meadows before tracking beside a small river.

I walked behind Brenda and my mom and spent the first ten minutes of our hike trying to figure out a way to gently broach the topic. But what sounded like an elegant suggestion in my head wound up lobbing through the air with a suddenness that even I wasn't prepared for.

"What happened when Mom got pregnant?" I asked.

My words landed on the ground in a rather gauche thud. This was followed by a slight lull in time—the three of us pausing so as to give my words a bit of breathing room.

"I mean . . ." I said slowly, in some attempt to recover. "I know *how* she got pregnant, but . . . what happened after that?"

"When I got pregnant?" asked my mom. "You mean with you?" She was slightly confused.

"No, Mom. When you got pregnant with Carl."

"Oh, with Carl."

Brenda turned back to look at me.

"I thought you might ask me about that," she said, before smiling her sparkly smile and starting in.

"Gosh, that was a long time ago. But I remember when Granny and Papa told me. I was . . . hmmm, I guess only about twelve or thirteen at the time."

She paused, and it was as if I could see her pulling in bits and pieces of the story.

"They sat me down," she continued. "I think Daph was already out of the house, maybe even married, and I don't remember Nancy being there."

We continued along the trail, a large stream of water appearing on our right. I noticed a handful of small, grey birds at the bank—American dipper probing for food underneath rock and stone.

"You know," said Brenda. "Nancy was still so young. Only seven or eight. I can't remember if she was there . . . if they even told her, but I remember them telling me that Sheila was pregnant. And I remember being so confused. 'But her and Brian aren't married,' I said."

Brenda stopped walking for a moment and laughed.

"That's how it was in our house, you know. We had no information. They told us nothing. I had no idea what sex was. I honestly thought the only way you could get pregnant was by getting married. Looking back, it's no wonder she got pregnant. We never talked about anything like that. Can you imagine Granny talking about the birds and the bees?"

We all paused on the trail for a chuckle. The answer was no. My grandmother, in all of her warmth, came with even fewer words than my mother.

Brenda continued on, and as she did, my mom started nodding along. It was as if the whole thing was actually jogging her memory enough that she could recall snippets here and there. On occasion she would even add something: "Yep, Brian." Or "Mhmmm. Papa was so good about everything, wasn't he? I told Papa first. Did you know that? I took the bus to his office."

"Yeah, I did, Mom. You told him there, right?"

"Yeah. Mhmmm," she said, nodding.

This was one of the only details I knew. We had been out for a walk, a year or so prior to our trip, and, in a similar fashion to what I had just done, she just blurted it out.

"I thought Granny would get too emotional," she said. "So I told Papa first. At his office."

As the conversation with my aunt continued, I felt a singular raindrop land on the top of my hand.

"I remember one day in July," she said. "I was at camp.

Granny and Papa knew the baby was coming, so they put us in camp. I think . . . I think Nancy was with me—anyway, I remember my counselor telling me I had to report to the office. I went, and when they held out a phone for me, it was Papa on the other end of the line. He told me that Sheila had her baby. Pretty soon after that I remember being back at home, at the house on McCleery Street."

"And what was it like?" I asked. "What was she like? Did she change?"

Brenda turned over her shoulder to look at me. Her face was sad.

"Yes," she said. "She definitely changed. That whole year. She was a different person. When we were young she had all this energy. She was cheeky—you know that—but the one thing I remember from that year was her in her room. She basically locked herself in her room for an entire year. She would just sit at her desk and do . . . what is it called? Paint by numbers. She just sat there and painted, colored. Every day for a year."

I looked at my mom.

She nodded.

"I colored," she said.

Part of me stood. And another part of me fell. I felt as though my whole stomach had been cut from some internal cord.

The number of things I don't know about my mother grows larger every day. It makes me feel lost, like I'm wandering aimlessly through the landscape of her life. I'm not even sure I know what I'm looking for anymore.

There was a long pause as we stood together on the hiking trail. It was my mother who broke the silence.

"I love coloring," she said.

"I know you do, Mom."

And there it was, snaking gently through the air, the scent of pencil shavings and juniper berries.

My mother stood alone in the wilderness of motherhood. In my mind's eye, I see her there. I see her arms outstretched and her hands held out. But they're empty. A baby boy quickly placed into the watershed on the other side of the divide. There was no one for my mother to mother.

I also imagine her exit. I imagine her being told it was time to leave and that she should never speak of what had happened. That it really would be best to never talk about where she had been, and to tell no one about what she had seen. I imagine that she was advised to leave it in the past, to build a door and close it, to forget about it. What this meant was that my mother wasn't even allowed to mother herself.

It's extraordinarily hard to heal a wound if the wound itself cannot breathe, is not acknowledged, is not even allowed to exist. It's close to impossible to heal a wound if the wound is bandaged up once and then forgotten. One might even say a wound like that is likely to fester, to rot, to travel by way of the blood so as to infect an entirely different part of the body.

My mother's first survival skill as a woman, as she crossed the threshold from maiden to mother, was to forget, and then, apparently, color the fuck out of things. It was the dam she built—forgetting, ignoring, and moving right on. It was the dam everyone and everything around her conspired to build.

They constructed it using an axe and bricks of erasure. It seemed no coincidence to me that now, as she made another transition, this one from mother to crone, she was reaching for and using the very same set of tools—the same shield and sword, the same set of thigh holsters.

The act of forgetting had delivered her once, and the pattern was about to repeat. It was clear to me now. Alzheimer's was going to deliver my mother. It was going to carry her from one place to the next, visiting the past so as to leap into the future. Since the moment she was diagnosed, since a year or two before that even, I had been watching my mother in the midst of jumping her own banks.

I didn't know whether to clap wildly for her, or collapse onto the stairs, slapping my hands on the rubber tread in protest.

11

Heartwood

*Someone decided a long time ago that naming
pain is impolite, that hiding it and hiding
from it makes more sense. It doesn't. It's a lie.
A lie that both comforts and destroys us.*

—SHONDA RHIMES

As we drove back to the campsite, the sky began the slow drop of its curtain. A thick, velvety dusk was settling in.

I turned to my mom and my aunt.

"Let's get a fire going as soon as we're back."

"I like that plan," my aunt said in agreement.

Shortly after, the three of us were circled around the firepit at our campsite. I handed my mom a few scraps of paper.

"Here you go, Mom," I instructed. "Crumple these up and then toss them in there."

"In here?" she asked, pointing toward a few pieces of charred wood and ash.

"Yep. Right there," I said, before pulling a few pieces of firewood out from under the picnic table.

"Will you hand me one of those?" asked my aunt, as she grabbed a small axe from the back of her car. "I'll make a bit of kindling."

I watched as my aunt began to rock the blade of her axe over a piece of wood, right along the edge—back and forth, back and forth, back and forth, until the steel was wedged into the wood. Once it was there, she lifted the axe in the air and brought it back down in an easy glide. The wood went along for the ride, and when it hit the ground there was a small thud followed by a satisfying clunk—the sound of the wood splitting off from itself. It seemed effortless, as if it never wanted to be attached in the first place.

My aunt, forever a student as well as a teacher, started in on a lesson.

"I'm learning all about this in my hiking group," she said. "When you run the axe with the grain, instead of against it, the wood just sort of falls apart. You have to position the blade in just the right place, and then—crack—a small piece will just pop right off."

As the wood split away from itself, I felt a kinship to it. I'd always felt that if I just got rid of that unnamed and unwanted part of myself, I'd fit in—like my belonging was contingent on chopping or slicing, on flicking away little droplets of water.

I watched my aunt repeat the motion seven or eight times, and each time she brought the wood back down to the ground, I felt a tremor rise up through my feet. I felt it course through my lower legs and up into my thighs until it reached my hips. It settled there, a dark and unnamable anger. I took a deep breath and grabbed the matches from the picnic table.

"I can't remember what it's called," said my aunt, her eyes fixed on the wood in front of her. "But someone told me the center wood is best. It's drier, I think."

"It's called heartwood," I heard myself whisper, as I watched another section of wood splinter off from itself.

"What's that?" my aunt asked.

"Heartwood," I said a little louder, anger seeping out from my cambium layer.

I was ten or eleven years old when my siblings and I were called to a formal family meeting. We'd never had such a meeting, and the only thing I knew about them (based on stories from my friends) was that they were almost always the precursor for divorce. I remember being instantaneously nervous.

We shuffled into the living room, and as we sat down, I made sure to grab a seat beside my brother Ryan. Every part of me wanted to be next to him. In that moment, my entire being was reliant on his buoyant energy, something to help lift me away from the large pit that was forming in my stomach.

My mother, who was almost always warm and steady and slow, seemed pulled in, gathered tightly at every hem. Her eyes were cast straight down. It was as if she was watching a giant river that had just appeared at her feet, perhaps wishing she could slip into it, perhaps hoping she would be carried right out of the room.

And then it happened. Before anyone even started to talk,

I watched my mother move in two directions at once. Part of her stayed seated; another part of her slid into the water and straight on out of the room. As she went, I felt a freeze set in, my insides getting colder and colder and colder.

I looked around the room. No one else seemed to notice she was gone. This made my insides even colder. In the space around me, I felt a flat kind of tension. We all sat stiffly, passing the tension around the room like a stone. I watched my brother pass it to my sister, and I watched my sister try to pass it to my mother. But my mother wasn't there, my mother could not take it, or hold it, or help us, not when she was busy swimming, trying to stay afloat. So my sister held it.

There's a chance she's been holding it every day since.

With the tension resting in my sister's lap, I felt myself reach for my brother. I clutched him energetically, while starting in on a frantic search for my mother.

Where is she? Where is she? Where is she?

There's a chance I've been searching every day since.

All of a sudden, I heard a handful of questions. They bounced around the room, furtive and quick. They came with small giggles.

Is this supposed to be joke-like? I wondered. I wasn't sure, but it made me feel better.

"Can we guess?" one of us asked. I don't remember which one.

"Are you getting a divorce?" asked another.

"Is Mom pregnant?" someone added.

I heard my dad's voice and quickly grabbed hold of it. It, too, made me feel better.

"That last one's pretty warm," he said, as he looked over at my mom. She still wasn't there.

Can he feel that? I wondered. *Does he know she's not here?*

He looked back to all of us.

"It's a close guess," he said. "But not exactly."

My dad continued on, filling us in on some of the details:

We were fresh out of high school.

We were in love but too young to get married.

The baby went to someone else.

A little later we got married and had all of you.

And now . . . we have the opportunity to find him.

He forged ahead. He painted a rather rosy picture. He told us some of the truth as my mother swam, or floated, or drowned, I'm not sure.

I don't remember how long we all sat there, but at some point my dad told us it was time for a breather.

"That's a lot to take in," he said. "Why don't we pause there?"

Pause, I wondered to myself. *But what about my questions?*

I was filled with questions:

Where is Mom?

Why am I so cold?

Would this new brother sleep at our house once we found him?

But I rarely, if ever, asked questions. There were three reasons for this. The first was that rosy pictures are wonderful, aren't they? The second was because Jaggers don't pry—we are agreeable creatures. And the third? Because if the youngest of four knows anything, it's that not knowing things is annoying, not cool, and inarguable proof of one's stupidity. I worked hard to demonstrate the opposite, to show my older siblings I knew just as much as they did, even when I didn't, even when it meant lying through my teeth.

And yet, as I look back through my life, I see that I had more questions. All of which had to do with being and becoming a woman, with the feminine. I know this because these questions cropped up at very particular times along the coming-of-age continuum.

I had questions about my mother, and about myself, as I inched toward puberty. I had more questions when I got my period for the very first time. Almost none of which were asked or answered. My mother's singular response to that particular event in my life was to tell me my sister had supplies in the bathroom upstairs. This was, quite literally, the only question I knew the answer to. But who would show me how to use the supplies? Who would talk to me about why the blood was so dark? Who would tell me what I was supposed to do at the birthday party next week, the one that included a trip to the Aquatic Centre on Beach Avenue? Who would tell me how to survive, now that embarrassment was such a consistent part of my life? Who would tell me this was, in fact, nothing to be embarrassed by? No one. No one would tell me these things.

I had lots of questions when I, at the same age as my mother had, started holding hands with boys, and kissing boys, and letting boys put their hands down my pants.

When I was sixteen I told my mother that some of my friends were on the pill and that maybe I should be too. We went to the doctor's appointment together. She sat in the chair in the corner of the room, and I sat on top of the crinkly white paper.

"Do you have any questions?" asked the doctor as she wrote up the prescription.

I looked at the blank face of my mom and then back to the face of the doctor—almost vacant and matter-of-fact.

"No," I said. "No questions."

This was a lie of epic proportions. Of course, I had questions. Couldn't they see them pouring right out of me?

I wanted to know what the pill would do to my body, and if the myth of bigger breasts was actually true. I wanted to know what would happen if I forgot to take a pill. And what if I forgot to take two? I wanted to know if my mom was going to go to the pharmacy with me, because Laura Biffen's mom worked at the pharmacy, and if she knew, and then Laura knew, and then everyone knew, I thought I might die. I wanted to know why some people used condoms instead of, or along with, the pill. I wanted to know if my mother had been on the pill and if she'd gotten pregnant anyway. I wanted to know how scared I should be. I wanted to know what the hell these two ladies were thinking as they sat there assuming the other one was going to fill me in on all this, somewhere down the road, somewhere in private. All the while I was left walking through a forest with forked paths toward my future, paths that went one way if I was armed with answers, paths that could go another if I was left without them. And I wanted to know why my mother wasn't telling me about the intimate knowledge she had about forks in the road.

As a little girl, I assumed that everything my father told

us that day in the living room, as well as everything my mom never said in addition, was part of a book called *All of the Truth*. As I got older, I realized I had misunderstood the title, and that the book was actually called *Part of the Truth*.

But what's the *Right Amount of Truth* to tell your children? Because surely, ten- and eleven-year-olds should hear different truths than seventeen- or eighteen-year-olds. And what, pray tell, does this mean about deciding upon the right amount of truth to tell ourselves?

As I got older, as I examined my own truths, one had become quite clear: I was angry with my mother. I was angry with her then, and I was angry with her now.

And this anger, its entrance was not obvious. It wasn't squirming around inside of me because of a singular event. Its arrival had been piecemeal, coming tucked into the pocket of every unasked and unanswered question. Over the years, it was wordlessly stitched into the lining of me. And when anger enters that way, you don't call it anger. In fact, you don't name it at all. You do what your mother taught you—you distance yourself from it and move on. You tell yourself you were well nurtured, and well cared for, because you were. And then you take a nap, because clearly you're tired.

You dismiss your own feminine nature—because you see how all of your unasked and unanswered questions center directly around it—and you label it small and non-valuable. And then, after a bit of time passes, you begin not to see it at all. You crack off any and all attachment to it. You develop an ego around not fitting the feminine mold, at the same time as maneuvering yourself into a different one, a more masculine one, one that doesn't quite fit but will do. You make yourself into something you're not. You become one of the guys. You go out of your way to prove that's what you are. You boast rather arrogantly about it. At least that's what I did.

I've often wondered about the swiftness with which I rejected the feminine. The ease with which I took up an axe. But really, there was nothing to wonder about at all. It was, after all, exactly what I was taught to do. My mother showed me how. And the world I grew up in, the society and the systems around me, they helped me to position the blade in just the right place.

Of course, there had been no clear lesson plan for this. It was a watch-and-learn kind of thing. I learned, through observation and osmosis, that hiding parts of myself, obscuring who I was, was both accepted and expected. When my father became the storyteller, I learned that the masculine voice carried more weight. When my mother kept parts of herself out of sight, I felt encouraged to do the same. And later, when I came to understand that everything my mother hid was not random, but connected to motherhood, to being and becoming a woman, I figured . . . well, the sooner you stop breathing life into something, the easier it is to cut it off. Because it's drier. Like heartwood.

I looked over to my mother, who was standing in front of a small pile of crumpled paper.

"What do we do next?" she asked.

I couldn't find words for an answer. My body was busy, now consumed by the anger. It felt as though all of the things my mother had never said, and perhaps never felt, were now in a bag, left for me to hold on to. Somehow, over the years, it seemed her pain had been transferred to me. And now, she would get to forget about it and move on, leaving the remembering part to me. This felt like a searing kind of thaw, and I didn't know what to do with the pain.

All of a sudden, I felt desperate to scream. The only problem being, I no longer knew how. I felt I might shatter, might turn into a pile of shards on the ground. My mind did not contain enough knowledge to know what to do with the hot, pumping pain in my feet, in my hands, in the tips of my fingers. I was not taught how to process this feeling. I was not taught how to feel it. In fact, I was taught that it didn't exist at all.

It was in that moment—matches in one hand, bag in the other—that I came to understand: there was more of me living outside of myself than there was remaining inside. My essence had been replaced with my anger.

Pain, in any variation, never did fit into the rather rosy family picture. It was very rarely shown and very rarely discussed. Space was not created in our household for anything other than silver linings, and the smell of rhubarb pie. I didn't know what to do with anger, nor had I a clue about how to handle sadness, sorrow, or unbridled rage. I didn't know where any of those things fit. They did not belong on the inside of me, but there they were regardless, and I didn't have a clue how to go about getting them out.

My first instinct was to yell at my mother. To grab her shoulders, to shake her, and howl. We had kept ourselves hidden from one another for so many years, and this was our final chance, for God's sake. Could she not see that?

But it was far too late for screaming. For to scream at a tiny woman with Alzheimer's would be pointless, and cruel to the both of us.

My second instinct was to turn it into heartwood. To pull all of it—the anger about my mother closing all those doors, and the rage about Alzheimer's locking them shut—further into my core, to hold it there for however long it took to run out of air. My instinct was to choke my anger with a vacuous darkness.

But this was an instinct I knew better than to obey. I sensed that the pain would continue to pulse through the bloodstream, to drum through us all, if I didn't bring it to the surface of me, to the surface of us.

"Pain travels through families," wrote transformational coach and mother wound healer Stephi Wagner, "until someone is ready to feel it."

I was not interested in sharing the same path as my mother, or her mother before her—an achingly slow dismemberment was a road I could not bear. And so I would have to figure out a way to bear the pain instead, to move it up and out of me, up and out of the soil I had grown from.

Heartwood is not the part of the tree that pumps water through the trunk, nor does it move sugar through the branches and limbs. It is not part of the vascular system of a tree. It is the opposite. Heartwood is composed of entirely lifeless cells. It is dead. It is the hardened evidence of what was. It is petrification at the core, at the innermost sanctum. A little bit of heartwood is fine. In fact, it helps to keep the tree standing. Too much of it, though, and the tree is at risk of rotting from the inside out.

The choice between feeling decades, perhaps centuries, of unfelt pain or attempting to survive inside a lineage that was being slowly erased was clear.

I would not pull my anger in. I had to find a way to pull it out.

I paused and looked up at the sky. As I did, a handful of memories popped into my mind. One after the other, a flip-book of my childhood and adolescence.

All the things by eight years old that I knew not to do. All the things by eleven I knew not to say. All the things by four-teen I knew not to be. The sound of wood splitting off from itself was ringing in my ears.

I have to figure this out, I thought to myself. *And I have no idea where to start.*

Beside me, I heard my mother repeat her question:

"What do we do next?" she asked in earnest.

"I don't know, Mom," I said. "I don't know."

My aunt struck a match and held it gently underneath the woodpile. The pieces of paper my mother had crumpled were the first things to catch fire. They carried the burn until the wood was ready to go. And then it all went up in flames—the incipient stage of a blaze.

I stood there watching the flames, hoping for a heat intense enough to melt everything inside that had frozen.

12

The Difference Between Erosion and Erasure

*It serves us well to turn our eyes earthward
and study the oft-overlooked wisdom beneath
our feet.*

—ROBERT MOOR

Our start the next morning was slow. I was tired and my mother was cold. I wrapped her in an extra down jacket and pulled our camping chairs over to the edge of Wild Creek, a meandering stretch of water that serves as the drainage for Saint Mary Lake. We lingered there, eating breakfast from that spot, watching the sun slide up the edge of the sky until it started casting light off the surface of the water.

As the sun rose, I noticed my mom starting to squint, so I walked back to the campsite and grabbed her sunglasses out of her purse.

"Put these on, Mom," I said, as I placed the sunglasses in her hands.

"Oooooh, that feels better." She sighed. "I forgot I had these. They're so handy, aren't they?"

I rested my hand on her shoulder and gestured for her and my aunt to hand me their dishes.

"Here," I said. "I'll get us cleaned up."

My mom handed me her mug and spoon before turning to my aunt.

"She's so talented," she said. "I don't know how she knows how to do all these things."

My aunt laughed, knowing full well it was my mother who taught me how to do most of the things I was doing.

"I'll take a bit more coffee," she added. "Only if there is some."

"Coming right up, Auntie B," I said.

As I walked across the small gravel easement, I heard my mom's voice.

"Look at those—"

She lost the word she was searching for.

"Dandelions," said Brenda, filling in the gap.

"Dandelions," repeated my mother. "Yes. They're all wearing funny yellow hats."

I looked over my shoulder, spotting the patch of yellow flowers my mother was looking at. They were sitting quite close to a bank of bright green clover. Dandelion is one of the fifty-some odd words removed from the Oxford Junior Dictionary in 2007.

Others that went with it include kingfisher, lark, otter, raven, starling, and thrush. Ash, bramble, holly, fern, and mint. Blackberry went too. So did clover. As the story goes, none of these words were used enough to warrant inclusion.

When I read about this, a lump the size of a chestnut formed in my throat. Chestnut is gone too, by the way.

The list of words that replaced the above were mostly technology based. Words like broadband, MP3 player, block graph, and chat room. As well as others like celebrity, debate, citizenship, and conflict. The two additions that stuck out the most, though, were the phrase "cautionary tale" and the word endangered.

This slow peeling away of words was also happening in my mother's brain. And for us as a collective, we're letting what seem like little things slip away, losing grasp of the words that quite literally make up the world around us. Forgetting them. What does this say about the world around us, I wonder? How fast will it slip from our fingers?

Later that morning, we threw a few granola bars and hard-boiled eggs into a pack, and we hopped into the car. It was a short drive to Lake Sherburne and an even shorter walk from the car to the trailhead. The park ranger had told us about a gentle four- or five-mile hike called Redrock Falls, which seemed perfect for a midday meander.

I let my aunt take the lead, my mom following closely behind her. They chatted away as they walked, and I allowed myself to fall a few paces behind. I felt tired. Familiarly so. This was the pull of a lifelong pattern—as emotions crept toward me, my instinct was to grab my pillow and curl into bed for a nap. I tried my best to stay awake, to shake this feeling off as I walked so as to allow for others that wished to emerge.

The aspen-lined trail opened up here and there to astounding views of Fishercap Lake. There were two or three people in the distance, waist-high in the water. I watched as they cast a series of fly lines. The lines looked like something a spider would make, sparkling silk draglines arcing gracefully through the air.

We kept walking, moving in and out of the forest path. The sound of small bells could be heard ringing here and there, a sign of bear-cautious hikers somewhere nearby. As we got closer to the turnaround, the grade of the trail increased ever so slightly and took us up through a meadow of low brush— huckleberry just starting to yield, and thimbleberry with fruit too pale to consider. It was too early in the season for anything sweet.

Up ahead of me, I noticed that my aunt and my mom had come to a stop. Once I caught up, I saw that they were taking in the views—Mount Wilbur, as well as Swiftcurrent Mountain, both considerable peaks in the Lewis Range.

As we continued on, I noticed the rock around us—it began shifting in color as we hiked higher in altitude. What had been light grey stone, streaked with chalky sulfur and speckled with pale green lichen, was becoming deeper and richer. It was taking on a purplish hue. By the time we got to the top the whole landscape was carmine—a red curtain of rocks with a small river running straight through the middle. It was a stunning rose-colored fountain with water cascading down shallow steps, moving in and out of an emerald-colored pool.

It was, quite literally, a rather rosy picture. And I was mad about it.

We sat for a bit, eating our granola bars and eggs. My aunt

showed my mom some of her favorite yoga poses. I picked up a handful of stones and threw them with force down into the water.

On our way back down the trail, about three or four hundred meters from the parking area, we came upon a small moose calf—all spindly-limbed and awkwardly cute. My mom began walking directly toward it.

"Here, moosey," she said, before making a slight sucking noise with her mouth.

"Mom!" I shouted as I began backing up off the trail.

To see a small animal in the wild—a baby cub, or a calf, or a pup—is a dangerous thing. Because right behind a baby is its—

"Mom!" I screamed.

She turned her head to look at me, and as she did I saw the mother moose standing there, staring at my mother. This moose was magnificent, and at the very same time, absolutely terrifying. My auntie Brenda grabbed the back of my mom's jacket and started pulling her backward.

My eyes were still on the moose, and the moose's eyes were, rather unfortunately, still on my mother. If you had asked me prior to that moment, I would have assumed that being stared at by a moose was much like being stared at by a deer. It is not. It is the opposite of that. A deer stares at you in an "I'm gonna freeze for a few moments here before I move into flight" kind of way. A moose stares at you in an "I'm gonna freeze for a few moments before I charge you" kind of way. It is extraordinarily frightening.

"Sheila," whispered my aunt. "Get. Off. The trail."

All three of us skittered to the edge of the path, ducked under a bit of brush, and, rather quickly, tiptoed the long way round to the parking lot.

Brenda and I, while in awe, were both quaking. My mother, on the other hand, was displaying zero evidence of fear. If anything she was more frustrated than scared.

"Why did you pull me?" she asked Brenda sharply. "I wanted to see the moose."

"No, Sheila," said my aunt, laughing. "No, you did not."

Once back in the car, we hooked onto a road that took us a bit further south. Before long, we pulled into a large parking lot behind the Many Glacier Hotel—one of the places in the area known for its breathtaking views.

We walked along the rocky shoreline of Swiftcurrent Lake and down onto the wooden docks, where a series of colorful canoes were being stored—locked but ready for action in the coming weeks and months. We were visiting early in the season; combine that with the fact that the previous winter and start of spring had been colder than normal, and there was barely another person around.

"I'm going to look for a bathroom," said my aunt. "She, do you want to come with me?"

My mom nodded. She looked a little cold.

"I'm gonna take a few photos," I said. "I'll meet you inside in a minute."

"Sounds good," said my aunt, before turning to my mom. "Let's go get you warm, She!"

I watched them as they walked quickly off the dock and up toward the hotel.

Once alone, I took a deep breath and let out a large sigh. As I did, I felt a few ripples of tension release from my shoulders. There hadn't been many moments on the trip where I had not been standing or sitting or sleeping right beside my mother. My mother, who, in this moment, I was mad at. Sort of. It was all so confusing.

Who am I actually mad at? I wondered.

I looked up at the mountains that rose steeply from the other side of the water. Mount Grinnell, a massive triangular peak, was in the foreground, as well as Mount Gould, a formidable mountain standing in the near distance. Like the peaks we saw that morning, these two were also part of the Lewis Range.

All of them were staggering—dramatically steep, sharply edged, gorgeously layered rock. They aren't as tall as many other peaks, especially those in their mother range, the Rockies, but they were just as striking. The shapes that they'd been carved and pushed into made them look like black diamonds rising straight from the earth.

The multiple glaciers in the area were hard to spot from where I was standing, but I knew they were there, all of them strung across the collarbones of those mountains like giant diamond necklaces—Grinnell Glacier and Salamander among them. Aprons of ice and giant, frozen rivers that have sliced through Glacier National Park, helping it to become the mountainous gem that it is.

I had read a bit about Glacier before we arrived, and the National Park Service had a quote on their site that said that all of the park's glaciers will be gone by 2030. They will have melted. They were doing so right in that moment, as I stood on the dock beside those colorful canoes. The glaciers, tucked here and there, just out of sight, were melting. They were disappearing, even on a freezing cold day in late spring.

When we lose something, we're usually only aware of it after the fact. A wallet. Our keys. Our favorite pen that we swear we used just this morning before putting it back on our desk. It's very rare for us to be conscious, to be awake to the fact that we are in the midst of the loss. We don't see ourselves losing our wallet, or our words, bit by bit—we don't go through our day knowing it's coming or watching it happen.

Most of the time, losing things doesn't really happen that way. Or maybe it does but it's just too hard a thing to look at, too hard a thing to bear.

Because losing something is one thing. But to be in the midst of losing it—to be in some liminal place, betwixt and between, where you must watch the thing as it goes—is a whole other story. I can't think of something harder to lock eyes with. I can't think of a single thing I would rather not see, never mind feel, and then have to remember.

During my first year of university, I thought of my mother almost every single day. She had only been a month or so into her own postsecondary education when she got pregnant, when she was all but forced to drop out.

In my first semester, as part of my leaning toward an arts education, I took a social work class. And when we were given topics to research, I chose adoption. It was the perfect excuse.

Finally, I thought to myself. *I'll get to ask all of my questions.*

I drafted a list. I made plans for how, under the guise of scholarly research, I could ask every question, every unknown that I was dying to know.

I phoned my parents' house during the day, when I knew my mom would be the only one home. And then, finally, I summoned the courage required.

"Where did you go?" I asked. "Like, do you remember the place you were sent when you were pregnant with Carl?"

My mother came up empty—entirely so. On that question and every other question I asked. She had not a single answer. She didn't know exactly where she went or who else was there. She wasn't sure what she wore or if she had a room-mate. She didn't know what food was served, or if she was allowed to use the phone. She didn't know how she got to the hospital, or if anyone had been there to hold her hand. Noth-ing, zip, nada, zilch. It was almost as if *All of the Truth* had simply dissolved before her very eyes. Perhaps it had been far too much to see, never mind feel, and then have to remember.

It was decided—how and by whom I don't know—that my mother would go to a house for unwed girls. Most people I've talked to, and most things I've read, refer to these places as "homes," but I won't. A home does not feel like a hospital–cum–cold church basement. A home, especially one for girls, doesn't forbid female visitors. A home does not require that you change your name upon arrival so anyone who knows you in here has no chance of knowing you out there. A home doesn't place an eighteen-year-old girl who just went into la-bor in the back of a taxi, with no information about what will occur when she gets to the hospital. A home doesn't use shame as a tool to silence people, to keep them in line. Or does it? I don't know anymore. I don't even know if any of the above fits with what my mother experienced and then promptly forgot—it was just part of the research I ended up doing for that social work paper.

What I do know is this: my mother was eighteen years old when she was encouraged to leave part of herself behind. To forget it and move on. And she was a month shy of her sixty-eighth birthday when she was diagnosed with Alzheimer's.

Fifty years is a long time to practice forgetting.

Fifty years. It's about the same amount of time it takes a fallen tree to disappear—after the wound occurs, after the fungus has traveled to the heartwood, and the rot has worked its way from the inside all the way out. After it sends any nutrients remaining back into the soil. From the moment the tree falls, to its full decomposition—fifty years. I read somewhere that red oak takes forty-nine years; balsam fir takes longer—a little more like sixty-three.

It will take the glaciers between ten and one hundred years to disappear. But they'll be gone too. And then what?

Will we still call it Glacier National Park when it no longer has any glaciers?

Will I still call her my mother when she no longer knows she has daughters?

What words will be swept off the pages of our dictionaries? Will anything be left? Will anything remain?

I stood on the edge of the dock and looked down at the water. I wished I could unlock one of the canoes and climb in.

And then, rather suddenly, my daydream was cut short. A reflection in the water caught my eye—a perfect halo of upside-down mountains was being cast back to me. Tears began rolling down my face as my eyes skimmed across the lake. I drank in the shimmering image that was being reflected—granite towers painted delicately on the surface of the water.

Look up, a voice whispered.

It didn't matter where the voice came from. I did as I was instructed and looked toward the sky, toward the mountaintops soaring in the distance.

Isn't it beautiful, what the ice revealed to us after it went cutting for stone? the voice asked.

I felt more tears slide down my face. With my gaze cast upward, I became suddenly sure the voice I was hearing was Mother Nature's.

The story doesn't lie in what's gone, but in what remains, it whispered. *You have to let one thing turn into something else, you have to let it transform—that's erosion. If you don't, my love—it will just go. And that's erasure.*

I felt myself wanting to argue. I mounted a defense.

"But that's not what my mothe—"

The voice cut me off.

Don't be so narrow-sighted as to think anything here has been erased, the voice continued. *Those mountains, and the rock that remains, they contain everything—minerals that serve as evidence of an ancient sea, colonies of fossilized algae, and sedimentary rocks that are almost a billion years old. There is ancient wisdom here. You might see something silent—just a large slab of stone—*

but don't go thinking a whole history, an entire way of being and knowing, doesn't reside deeply inside of it.

"But she didn't transfor—"

Shhhhhhh, said the voice. *Of course, she did. Just look back at the water and you'll see.*

Ever so slowly, from the edge of the dock, I looked back down at the water. In it was the liquid reflection of my very own face.

Those glaciers are my mother. The rock being revealed underneath them is me.

My mother let her pain turn into something else. She let it erode into a quiet and demonstrative kind of love. She surrendered. She let life carve something out of her. My mother's pain wore itself away, it ground itself down. It turned from rock into clay. And with that clay she made each and every one of us.

My mother is a sculptor, and her five children are the transformation of her pain. She surrendered many times over, not knowing who she might be on the other side of it all. And now, now I was watching her do it one more time.

Could I do that? I wondered. *Could I transform pain into love?*

I heard my aunt's voice from the shore and looked up.

"I thought you were going to meet us inside," she said. "I highly recommend those bathrooms—much more fancy than the bushes we've been using," she added with a laugh.

I quickly wiped my eyes and turned to face her. She was standing arm in arm with my mother, whose eye had already been caught by the same reflection, the series of images dancing on the water.

"Isn't it beautiful . . ." she said, her voice trailing off.

My mother is a mountain that was carved. A soul born big—a person who needed wind and water, fire and ice to sculpt it into formation.

I am a mountain that requires a push. A soul born small—a person who needs unearthing and upheaval, a soul that needs a shift in the fault lines for any rise at all.

13

Borrowed Landscapes

Whether or not we actually resemble the image we see, our mothers are our first, and most lasting, reflection of ourselves: a mirror we gaze into from birth until death.

—GLYNNIS MACNICOL

We spotted a diner on the side of the road. It was painted light purple and had a bright blue-and-orange sign on the side of it that read: TWO SISTERS.

"Well, we have to stop here," said my aunt, chuckling from the back seat of the car.

I pulled into the gravel lot, and the three of us walked inside.

We ordered club sandwiches and large baskets of french fries. And while we contemplated dessert, I used the diner's Wi-Fi to look up information about moose and what a sighting might symbolize on a spiritual level. I found a website describing various plant and animal meanings, and when I landed on moose, I read a bit of the description to my aunt and my mom:

"In spite of their huge size," I read, "they are able to move through their territory totally unseen. Moose teach us the power of presence and invisibility. They are wise, and balanced—knowing when to make their presence known, knowing what to say, when, and to whom."

"Sheila." My aunt laughed. "You're a moose! That explains everything—including why that moose decided not to trample you today!"

My mom raised her arms and placed her thumbs on either side of her head. Once there, she wiggled her fingers and stuck out her tongue.

"I'm a moosey," she said, between a fit of giggles. "Here, moosey, moosey."

My mother is a moose. Just because I didn't hear her doesn't mean she hadn't been there—talking, guiding, nudging, showing me all the various paths I could take. All this time I'd had her wrong. All this time I've had a lot of things so very wrong.

"Looks like you three are having fun," said our waitress as she slid a large serving of berry crumble across the table.

"We are," said my mom. "So much fun."

She reached for one of the dessert spoons.

"Is this my . . ."

She couldn't find the word.

"Spoon," I said. "Yep, that's your spoon."

"Oh good," she said. "That's what I thought. I needed to know which one was mine so you didn't steal all the pudding."

With that, she shot me a cheeky look and used her spoon to push mine out of the way, ensuring she had first dibs.

When the three of us were finished with the crumble, the bowl looked clean enough to be placed directly back in the cupboard—a clear sign that a Humphrys woman has been at it. Impeccable table manners (including a strong command of the knife, fork, and spoon) combined with a love of sweets (bordering on gluttony) makes for a high level of efficiency when it comes to clearing any evidence of food from a dish.

On the way back to the car, Brenda pointed toward the TWO SISTERS sign.

"Let's take a picture," she said, gesturing for me to pull out my camera.

My mom looked up at the sign and was suddenly confused.

"But we're three sisters," she said.

"No, She," my aunt replied, as she threw her arm around my mom. "You and I are the silly sisters."

"Bu—"

"That's Steph," said my aunt. "That's your daughter, Steph."

My mom paused and then smiled at me.

"Steph," she said slowly, as if to conjure a memory or two. "Always in the basement with a book."

She stared at me for a few moments longer.

"You . . . you turned out so pretty," she added, as if I was still young and somehow she'd snuck into the future to catch a glimpse of me.

Alzheimer's is my mother's theory of relativity. It's a coiling of time. It is the past and the present and the future at once—a wormhole, an Einstein–Rosen bridge. One day soon it will all collapse. One day soon she will disappear within it. But if you believe that everyone around you has already disappeared, does it even matter?

Whenever I look at the picture I took that day, the one of my mother and aunt in front of that restaurant, I wonder if it is in fact them, or if it is Picasso's *Two Sisters* from 1902, or Renoir's from 1881. Or perhaps, I think to myself, perhaps it's Mother Nature's—the Twin Sisters of the Cascade Range, formed in the Mesozoic era.

It wasn't the first time my mother had been confused about who I was. A confusion that started well prior to our trip and continued, with ferocity, throughout.

On the morning of our flight, the two of us had been standing in the upstairs hallway of our family home. I had just walked out of the bathroom, and there she was, about to head downstairs.

"Morning, Mom," I said.

"Oh!" she said. "Good morning."

She was slightly caught off guard, like she hadn't expected to see me, or perhaps to see anyone, in her house that early.

I paused for a moment to let her brain catch up, and when I thought it had, I looked into her eyes.

"I love you, Mom," I said.

"Thank you," she said, with a bit of surprise in her voice.

It was a peculiar response. The kind you would give if a stranger or kindly neighbor had just done you a simple favor—held the door open, for example, or stood to give you their seat on the bus.

She turned to head downstairs, and then, just before the first step, she swung around to face me.

"And I love you too," she said, before continuing down the stairs.

The second response was equally as odd as the first. Her tone was very matter-of-fact, like she knew she was supposed to say it but didn't know exactly why.

My mother knows she loves me, I thought to myself, *but she doesn't know why.*

There was no longer enough evidence in her brain about who I was, about the precise bonds we held, or the experiences we shared. There had been too much withdrawn from the bank. Love had turned from love to a common sense equation.

If this person is in the upstairs hallway of my house, and if they look familiar-ish, and are telling me they love me—well, that must mean we are related in some way, that must mean I love them, or, at the very least, am supposed to.

It would take another year or so before I was entirely fluid to her—the memory of me lapping gently against her shore.

Did she feel dizzy, I wondered, with the people in her life moving in and out, in and out, in multiple variations of themselves? Living in a place where time seemed to be fluid? Was it confusing—people sometimes appearing as they were in that moment, other times appearing as someone familiar whose name she just could not recall? And other times still, as an attentive stranger, a person she would turn to, and in a slightly panicked way say, "Oh my gosh! What time is it? I have to get home to the kids."

The word "remember" comes from late Latin, *rememorari,*

"to call to mind." My mother's brain could no longer do that, but in some strange way I felt her body could. And I wished there had been a word for that, an expression of some kind, another Latin phrase maybe.

There's implicit memory—all the things we remember to do without thinking about them—as well as explicit memory—the conscious recollection of things. The French have a term—*mémoire-habitude*—used to describe something more akin to muscle memory, the body's memory of a repeated action. But I wanted a different word.

On some level, I felt her knowing of me was no longer an action her body knew how to do, but rather a feeling her body knew how to feel. Something somatic. I felt as if her body's knowledge of me was cellular—a wordless recognition that ran across every inch of her, right underneath her skin, a fascial remembrance.

But then that was gone too. Another year or so passed and I had all but vanished. Extinct from my mother's mind, all traces of me expunged from her body.

Was it cold in that place, where everything you knew had up and disappeared? Was it terribly lonely? And what happens to those who are forgotten? The unremembered?

As my mother forgets who I am, I worry that I'll forget too. That my identity, the one I felt I was just coming to know, will ebb further and further away.

A lot of people say that when someone we love dies, a piece of us goes with them. But as I zipped my mother into her sleeping bag later that night, I wondered if they might be wrong. I wonder if what they really mean is that when someone we love dies, they're not around to reflect our identities back to us anymore. It feels like a piece of us is suddenly missing, when in actual fact, what we are being called to do is muster the strength and courage required to reach down and grab the mirror our loved one was holding on our behalf.

I wonder if we could do that. And if we could, I wonder if we'd see ourselves there, whole, shining back as brilliantly as ever.

I found this hard to believe, especially when it comes to our mothers.

Who am I without her? I wondered to myself, as I tucked her into bed that night, placing my head on the pillow beside her.

To know the interior of someone, to have lived inside of them, to have experienced all of them, to have been bathed in their every thought, in their every emotion—we can only say this of our mothers. Our existence is formed by way of swimming in the consciousness and unconsciousness of our mothers. Our hearts take a rhythm based off of theirs, our minds form like a palmar grasp holding firm to their wishes and worries. Knowing a person in this way makes it close to impossible to pull apart what is theirs and what is ours, to understand who and what we are, separate from them.

My mother is the landscape beneath and inside of me; she has held me from underneath since before time was time. She is the rock and loamy soil I have grown from, been nurtured by. And somehow, somewhere along the way, I became convinced that what she had given me was mine, when in fact, all along it had been borrowed, a landscape on loan. And I am terrified to give back what I have borrowed from my mother, because, Dear God, who and what will remain?

I listened to my mother breathing beside me. It was a slow and steady rhythm. I was tempted to lay my head on her chest, to feel it as it moved up and down, to synchronize my heartbeat to hers, but I didn't want to wake her. Or perhaps I didn't want to wake myself. Not now. Not just yet. Waking up to it all felt so hard.

She was vanishing just like those glaciers. I could see it happening when I looked at her, when we were standing face-to-face as well as in the photos I took. There was a slackening occurring, a very subtle softening of her jaw. And her eyes, the light was fading from behind them. Her nutrients were being leeched from the heartwood back into the soil. She was emptying. And I don't know what I will do when she's gone. There will be no mirror. There will be no map.

I reached into the tent pocket for my phone. I turned it on, opened the camera app, and toggled it to selfie mode. And then I lay there looking into the grainy image of myself being cast back by the phone. In the relative darkness, I began searching for her face in my own. I stared. I touched my cheeks and the tip of my nose. I traced the lines that had, a few years back, started running across my forehead.

Are these lines like her lines? I thought to myself. *Are her cheeks in my cheeks?*

I don't think we look very much alike, she and I. I don't think we are very much alike. I do have her exceptionally small feet and slightly crooked hips. I carry her worry within me like a heavy stone. But I cannot see her face. Her small, crystal-colored eyes, the smile lines that move out and up from the edges of them. Her button nose and short forehead, her clean jawline and warm, rosy skin. I cannot see it or feel it. I cannot sense her in anything I see in myself.

As I lay there in that tent, I felt a sudden groundlessness. As if there was nothing to hold me. Nothing from below. Nothing from above. Nothing even from within.

I lowered the phone. I felt dizzy. The whole world was spinning around me like some kaleidoscopic reality.

Do I even know who I am? I thought.

My mind frantically flipped through memories—all the times in the last few months when I stood in front of my mother, watching her take me in while searching herself for who, exactly, I was. All the times I stood there rocking on my feet—heel to toe, heel to toe, heel to the tip of my toe—waiting for the moment she named me.

Who am I if I am not my mother's daughter? I wondered. *Who am I if not the girl pushing back against her?*

In the whirling darkness of the tent, I felt something move in, some possibility inside of the spinning.

Perhaps this is it, I thought to myself. *Maybe her forgetting me is a gift.*

It only took a few moments for this to click into place. And when it did, the swirling—it suddenly stopped.

If my mother forgets who I am, I too am allowed to forget, to let go of who she sees me as, so as to focus on who I am becoming.

If my mother no longer recognizes me, I have permission

to do the same. I have permission to go back and pick up my essence, all those droplets of water I flicked away. And after that, I have permission to rush forth, with my wholeness, to be and become all the things that I hear calling.

Imagine what's possible if we let go of ourselves—the masks we've worn, the roles we've played, the performative nature of who we've become. Imagine if we were able to glimpse some unrecognizable future and run for it, no expectations, no decades-long narrative—ours, or our mother's, or anyone else's—holding us back?

As I lay there in the darkness of the tent, a sensation rushed through my body—some bullwhip of energy shot from the top of my head all the way down to my toes and back up again. This felt like a reclamation and reinvention at the same time. Or at least the possibility of it.

A silver thread had made its way into the lining of our story. For the minute my mother began to forget who I was, was the minute I could begin to remember.

I felt my tiny hand unfurl. I felt myself let go of her finger.

I hadn't a clue what came next, but it didn't seem like a coincidence to me that all of this clarity had come in the dark, in a womb made of night sky and nylon, nothing but the sound of my mother breathing beside me as she slept. I had a feeling my passage through life might be like that forevermore—wayfinding in the darkness, the shadows around me as a template to trace from. Running my hands along the side of the wall so as to find a path forward. The chorography of my interior. Artfully mapping the thousand miles of wilderness that my mother planted inside of me in the days before I was born.

This journey was never about me as seen through my mother, or my mother as seen by me. This was about an allowance—the two of us providing an expanse for one another, space to be who we have been, and had been, all along. This was a divinely feminine act, both the gift of the space and the notion that a rebirth, a grand transformation, could take place within it.

This was the feminine in all of her glory—the ability to birth all that has been withheld. To transform. To unearth a wild essence. A rebirth of self, so as to stand in the fullness of our nature.

And in that moment, I started to understand my mother's silence, the things she had held for her and her only. After finding her own internal map, pathways of transformation and deliverance, it's no wonder she guarded them. For this was the holy grail of her own alchemy.

My mother knew, as a good alchemist knows, that if anything is to be gained from the fire, something must be given to the flames. And I had not yet given a thing.

My mother is an alchemist, a mystic. Alzheimer's is her philosopher's stone. Forgetting is some long, winding trail toward remembrance, for her and for me, perhaps for us all.

As I lay in the tent, I felt some part of my landscape cleave off and slide, a small piece of my anger melting away. Just before I went to sleep that night, I felt a certain clarity settle inside of me: this trip was never about unearthing the mystery living inside my mother, but the one that has been living deep inside of me.

14

A Flag of Surrender

*Sadness does not sink a person; it is the energy
a person spends trying to avoid sadness that
does that.*

—BARBARA BROWN TAYLOR

Tears fell down my mother's face as she watched her sister's car pull away from the campsite. When we could no longer see it nor hear it somewhere around the bend, my mother turned to face me. She didn't say anything. She just stood there looking at me, rare evidence of her sadness still shimmering wet on her cheeks.

About an hour later, we pulled away from the campsite ourselves. Down the gravel road, and back onto the winding mountain highway—this time headed south.

The mountains on the western side of Glacier National Park spike, up and down, until they melt into the ocean. They are Mother Nature's cardiogram. The mountains on the east side are different. They come to a hard stop. The Lewis Range and the Rocky Mountain Front close out abruptly, a tightly tapered waist that marks the beginning of the Great Plains—specifically, the Northern Great Plains, a long grassy steppe that stretches across the rest of the state of Montana and well on into North Dakota. I wasn't accustomed to seeing that much land pulled out before me, an eyeful of it, a revelation.

As we dropped down into those grasslands, I was immediately struck with a strange sensation—a wild kind of peace infused with raw vulnerability, vulnerability that comes with exposure. Because while you can see everything that's out on the prairie, everything can also see you.

We hooked east and crossed over a small creek on our way to a town called Browning, the main community and seat of tribal government for the Blackfeet Nation. About two or three miles before town, a sign caught my eye. I couldn't read all of it, but I saw a painting of a yellow tipi and the word "gallery" written up above it. On top of the sign, there was a white flag fluttering in the breeze.

As I drove, the image of that flag stayed with me, gently flapping in my mind's eye.

Before long we pulled into Browning for lunch.

"Where are we going next?" asked my mom after we ordered some food.

"Good question," I said. "I'm not quite sure."

Our original plan had been to drive north, across the Canadian border, for a loop through Waterton Lakes, Banff, and Kootenay National Parks. But after looking at the road reports and weather conditions, I decided against it. Most of the roads were still covered in snow, and the temperatures were too chilly to camp with the gear we had. Add to all of that the fact that my mom was already cold for 75 percent of our waking hours, and our loop north was a no-go.

Although I knew I would have to come up with an idea of where to go next, I also knew we were in no rush to be anywhere.

"Why don't we take a look," I said, while reaching into my bag for the regional guidebook that was inside, something we could flip through for ideas. But as my hand searched for the book, the image of that white flag popped back into my head.

Surrender, I thought to myself. *A white flag means surrender, a truce before collecting the wounded.*

"You know what, Mom—I think there was an art gallery a while back on the road. I want to stop in there," I said. "And then I think we'll head back south, to Helena or something, maybe spend a night in the city."

My mom smiled.

"Sounds nice," she said, while nodding her head.

We paid our bill, hopped back in the car, and within a few minutes I saw the flag and slowed down so I could read the sign underneath it:

LODGEPOLE GALLERY
TIPI VILLAGE

We pulled into the long driveway and made our way toward a series of buildings—what looked like a main house and a handful of other small structures. There was a slight incline to the road, and as we drove up it the field below was revealed.

Ten or twelve tipis spilled out onto bright green grass. A handful of them were painted, but most were stark white—sparkling like stars on a green frontier, with the crisp blue Montana sky hung boldly in the background.

"Where are we?" asked my mom softly. Her words were spoken in the same cadence and tone as the opening of a fairy tale—once upon a time, somewhere long ago, there used to be a place.

"I'm not really sure," I responded. "How 'bout we ask?"

The two of us got out of the car and walked toward the house.

I knocked gently on what seemed like a side door.

"Hello . . . ?" I said, announcing our arrival.

From the outside, it was hard to tell if this was a gallery, or a house, or someone's private art studio. I was worried we might be in the wrong place, but then we heard a woman's voice calling out from a room further inside.

"Back here," said the voice.

As we continued inside, it became even more difficult to tell exactly what this place was. Each corner was filled to the brim with art—complete pieces and works in progress. We made our way past a handful of paintings, a selection of beautiful pottery, some animal hides decorated with beads and feathers, and a few racks of hand-painted greeting cards.

Just around the corner we found another room full of art. And toward the back, I saw a woman sitting behind a desk. She was quietly sorting through some papers.

As we walked closer to her, she paused, looked up, and smiled.

"Wow," I said. "Is all of this yours?"

I was referring to the art.

"Most of it's Darrell's," she said, standing up from her chair. "But we have a lot of other local artists as well. Feel free to snoop around."

"Thanks," I said. "We will. And who's Darrell? Should we know who Darrell is?"

"He's my husband," she said. "Well-known Blackfeet artist."

I nodded along as she spoke.

"I was just going to get up and make some coffee," she said. "Would you like any?"

"Oh, we just had some at lunch," I said. "But thanks."

The woman left the room and came back a few moments later, steaming mug of coffee in hand.

"You just passing through?" she asked.

"Yes. Well . . . sort of," I said. "We—"

My mom was standing beside me, so I wrapped my arm gently around her.

"This is my mom," I said. "We were just in Glacier for a few days and we were supposed to head north for a bit—but gosh, it's still so cold up there."

"Cold here too," she said. "Winter seems to be holding on this year."

"Exactly," I said. "So we're adjusting our plans. I'm not sure where we're headed next. Maybe Helena for the night."

"You should stay here," said the woman.

"Sorry . . . what do you mean 'stay here'?" I asked.

"Here," she said, gesturing for us to follow her out the back door.

We walked outside through a door at the back of the house. From there, an even more impressive view of the tipis was revealed.

"You can stay in one of these for a night," she said, pointing toward the tipis.

She led us back inside.

"You're on Blackfeet land," she instructed. "You should stay awhile. We serve dinner too. Darrell makes traditional recipes. Tonight is a meat stew."

"What do you think, Mom?" I asked.

She didn't say anything. She didn't have to. She was still staring wistfully in the direction of the field full of tipis.

We paid for one night's stay and went back to the car to grab our sleeping bags and camping chairs. After that, the woman, whose name we discovered was Angelika, led us toward a row of tipis at the bottom edge of the field. As we walked, I noticed prairie dogs poking their heads out of small burrow holes all around us.

"Any of these are great for two people," said Angelika, pointing to a handful of options. "And everything you need is inside—kindling, firewood, matches, and a few blankets for you to put over your sleeping bags. Darrell will serve dinner around six."

"Sounds great," I said.

Angelika walked back up the small hill, and I turned to my mom.

"How about this one?" I asked, as I lifted a large canvas

flap on the side of one of the tipis. Once inside, we found ourselves in a space large enough for us to stand in, which felt luxurious compared to our tent. There was a small firepit in the center, and although there was enough room to sleep three or four people, there were two obvious sleeping areas set to the outer perimeter of the tipi—blankets piled just so in the grass. A stack of pre-chopped wood had been set off to the side.

I looked up to the top of the structure. Canvas and poles, circled and gathered in such a way so as to reveal a small opening in the middle, a place for the smoke to escape and starlight to stream in.

We rolled out our sleeping pads and bags and I turned to my mom. "Do you want to color?" I asked. "I wouldn't mind getting our camping chairs out so we can sit in the sun."

The temperatures were still cool, but the sky was wide and clear, the sun high up in it.

"Color what?" she asked.

"Here," I said, pulling her coloring book out of her bag and handing it to her. "Let's set up the chairs."

"What chairs?" she asked.

"These ones," I said, as I grabbed our two camping chairs and ducked back out of the tipi.

"Come on, Mom," I called to her from outside.

While I assembled her chair, I noticed more prairie dogs. They were popping in and out of their holes, sometimes darting across the field to a different opening in the ground.

I heard my mom's voice.

"This is so neat," she said, as she popped her head out of the tipi. "I can't tell if this is a house or a room. Are we sleeping here?"

"We sure are," I said, while pointing at her chair. "Here, Mom. Come sit beside me and color."

"Color what?" she asked.

I laughed.

"The book," I said. "The one in your hand."

She stepped out of the tipi and looked at the coloring book in her hand.

"Oh, this," she said. "I was wondering what this was."

She sat down in her chair and placed the coloring book in her lap.

"Do you want your pencils?" I asked.

But she didn't answer. She just stared at the field in front of her, a smooth lake of green grass. She smiled, and after staring out for some time she shifted and held her face up to the sun.

As I was setting up my chair, it occurred to me that, for the first time on this trip, we would not be camping on public lands. I wasn't sure if Darrell and Angelika owned the land we were on, or whether they leased it, but it was clearly within the boundaries of the Blackfeet Indian Reservation.

I sat back in my chair, my mother at my side, both of us staring at the fiercely blue sky up above us, an ocean of grass at our feet.

The concepts and definitions of public land and private land, stolen land and indigenous land snaked together in my brain. *We do this with land,* I thought to myself. *We map it,*

and claim it, and mark up who owns it. But we do this with
people too. Because who are we if not the holders of this or that
or them?

My family has only had a few collective conversations about
my mother—about the loss being thrust upon us, about what
was happening, what could or would happen, or how quickly
things would go. We moved around those conversations delicately. We performed a maypole dance on a ground made of
eggshells.

And none of those discussions, not a single one, ever included my mother's voice. I've always wondered if she and my
father talked about those things in private. I wondered if they
made decisions as a pair about what she needed and wanted,
about what he needed and wanted, about lines in the sand of
their marital vows, or if either of them were scared. It didn't
seem so, but I didn't know for sure.

Needless to say, my family was ill-prepared for conversations that went beyond rosy pictures and silver linings. None
of us wore shades of grey with very much grace.

I remember being gathered together on a patio one summer night. We were sitting around a large oval-shaped
table—my siblings, a handful of our spouses, and my father,
the mourner in chief. Emotions ran high. The eggshell par-
quet was especially elaborate. And we had not practiced the
choreography.

At one point in the evening my father got defensive—hard
not to when grief, disguised as the thoughts and opinions of

five or six people, is moving at you with speed. As siblings and spouses, we made up a collective. As a parent, my dad was alone. He pushed back at us, after what comment by whom I cannot remember.

"Look," he said tersely. "I'm losing my wife. I'm gonna be losing my babe."

The underlying message was clear. He was losing something we were not. His stake was different than ours.

I can still hear my sister's voice in response, trembling but firm.

"And I'm losing my mother," she said.

The underlying message was clear. She was losing something he wasn't. Her stake was different than his.

Both of them were right. As author and grieving expert David Kessler has said, the worst loss is always our own.

The conversation went jerkily on from there. This was us, doing our best to love one another round and round the maypole. Looking back, I see we never needed a conversation, but communion in its place. We needed to learn how to feel, how to minister to ourselves and then to one another. We still need to learn this.

When I woke up the next morning, I couldn't stop thinking about this—the fact that everyone was losing something that someone else was not.

My father, his wife.
My sister, her mother.
My brothers, the very first woman who had them
   and held them.

My aunts, a steady stone, a full quarter of what
comprises their pack.
My mom's best friends, their quiet, but often
goofy, confidante.
The children of my siblings, the grandmother who
laughs and plays with them from ground level.
Me, the topography of my identity, the landscape
of my interior.

Grief can be a surveyor, someone who comes in to draw up
the property lines. And we were staking our claims. A roll of
flagging tape was being run from one corner of my mother,
diagonally, all the way across to the other side of her. I knew
this because I was caught holding one end of it.

We were each beginning to narrow our focus, to see nothing but our unique losses. We were donning grief-based vision
that highlights what is being taken from you and blinds you
from seeing what others are losing. And when one looks at
the world around them that way, the next question—even if
unheard, even if unseen and unspoken—comes in like poison
in the groundwater.

"If something is being taken from you," it whispers, "surely
that means that something is owed."

I thought my mother's story was mine to have and to hold.
I felt as though it was owed to me, like I had some sort of en-
titlement, a deed to *All of the Truth*. I felt as though this was
my inheritance. After years of her holding it in, my sense of
loss seemed to be demanding, begging really, that she hand it
over, lay it all bare on the table. I was desperate—because, in

the words of novelist Richard Powers, "things are going lost that have not yet been found."

What I didn't understand in those moments, in the days we spent dancing around the maypole, was that yes, everyone was losing something different—but it didn't really matter because all of us were losing.

It was plain and clear. We were a whole group of people hunched over inside of ourselves, shuffling slowly through the pain, at the very same time pretending it wasn't there. Unable to bear our own sadness. Because we'd grown up being agreeable, thinking it was best to move away from our pain, it was hard to accept any loss, to stop the rather delicate dance and watch as something like her slips from the palms of our hands. Instead, we each made our claims, and held on until our knuckles turned white, until our nails made marks on the insides of our hands. All because we never learned the difference between loss and defeat and surrender. All because we were never shown that after death comes rebirth.

My mother and I ate salted meat stew while watching the sun set on the edge of the earth. After dinner we moved into the tipi, and I built a small fire in the center. Around seven thirty my mom snuggled down into her sleeping bag.

"It's so warm in here," she said.

I nodded, while reaching for another log, and when I looked back, my mother was sound asleep. Her hands like soft paws, resting in the space between her cheek and the edge of her makeshift pillow.

A whole river of images rolled through my mind. Memories of my mother sleeping. Her feet up on the armrest of the couch, running shoes still on, slightly slack-jawed on a Sunday afternoon. My mother splayed out on a chaise lounge deck chair after a day of springtime gardening. Her legs in the shape of a V, her arms resting gently at her side—savasana pose years before she started going to yoga. My mother again, when I was a teenager—I would wake early for morning track practice. Before I left, I'd walk down the hallway and peek into her room. Her clothes from the day prior, as well as her worry, would be folded neatly on the chair beside her dresser. She would put them both on again soon, but for now, there she was, curled on her side, face softly smooshed by the pillow underneath her.

Without me realizing it, these had been my mother's first lessons to me in surrender, her ability to press pause on the world around her, to claim rest. They were white flags fluttering in the breeze. As I watched her sleep in the tipi that evening, I understood there had been many such lessons. And that this moment, too, was a lesson, but somehow it seemed different than the rest. Perhaps it was the crackling fire. Perhaps it was the ribbons of smoke moving through the air. Regardless, I felt ready for the initiation, ready to walk through my own alchemical fire.

How did I become so convinced that all of this was mine? I wondered. *How did I come to believe she owed her whole self to me?*

All of a sudden I felt my feet hit the shore. I was ready to return to my mother. To return, and see her off, all in one go. To stand on the shoreline wholly myself.

As I closed my eyes that night I felt something slipping, slipping through the palms of my hands. Me letting go of what I thought my mother owed me. Me letting go of that brightly colored flagging tape, the ribbon I had held as I moved around the maypole.

I had to feel my sadness. I had to let the anger I carried about the long, slow loss of my mother burn through to the hot coals at the center of me—the rage I carried about the loss of myself. The closed doors, the pathways toward femininity, hers and mine both, almost entirely blocked. The subsequent inaccessibility to our wholeness, the ability to hold on to the entirety of our essence. I had to move through all of that to find what was on the other side. I had to let go of what I thought I was owed, so as to move into oneness, a place of wholeness, where everything belongs, both sound and glorious silence.

My focus shifted away from the loss. It felt, now, that there was much to be gained.

15

A Place Called Wisdom

I woke in the middle of the night. I could feel cool air seeping in from under the edge of the tipi. I peeked, my eyes half-closed, and saw that the fire was all but extinguished, just a small pile of glowing red cinders. Although I was still warm in my sleeping bag, I knew I needed to get the fire going again for things to stay that way. With much reluctance, I crawled out of my sleeping bag, stirred the embers, and reached over to the pile of wood for another log or two.

As I was crouched, tending the fire, I glanced across to the other side of the tipi. The light was dim, but I could see my mother's face, the outline of her body moving gently up and down as she breathed. My sweet mama, sound asleep in the same position she first dozed off in.

I started moving back toward my sleeping bag, but before I wriggled in, I thought maybe I should go outside and find a place to pee.

I'm already up, I thought to myself. *And I don't want to have to get out of my bag again.*

I slipped my feet into the pair of running shoes I'd placed at the foot of my sleeping bag and tiptoed toward the door of the tipi. I raised the flap to one side, stepped out, and quietly rolled it back down behind me.

Once outside and away from the fire I couldn't see a thing. I hadn't brought my headlamp on this midnight excursion, and I immediately regretted it. Everything around me was black. It was as if I had been devoured, swallowed whole by the night's gaping jaws. If my pulse weren't there as some measure of myself, chanting inside of my chest, thrumming at my wrist and the side of my neck, I'm not sure I would have known I existed.

Even though I knew there was nothing in front of me, I instinctively raised my arms up into the air, my hands moving gently around in search of—I didn't know exactly. Something to hold me up? Something that might knock me over? I looked toward the ground. Again, blackness. Regardless, I kept my eyes there, crouched down a little for balance, and inched my way forward in the dark. I wanted to go as far from the tipi as was appropriate to pee, but not so far that I wouldn't be able to find my way back.

Why did I not grab my headlamp? I thought to myself.

Once I was some unknown distance out in the field, I pulled my pants down and moved into a low squat. It was then that I started to hear things that I could not see. I bounced back up, pants still at my ankles, wondering if I should make a dash back to the tent. Was that the noise a prairie dog made at night? Was that a coyote in the distance? Or was it just the bray of a horse coming from a neighboring field? My heart was racing.

"Stop," I said to myself, in a firm but whispering voice. "There is nothing here that wasn't here in the day. Just pee and go back to bed."

I did as I instructed.

When I was finished, I pulled my pants back up and stood tall, looking now to the sky. Why I hadn't done so prior was a mystery to me. The sky was completely clear. So clear it seemed I could see every star in this galaxy, and perhaps even the next.

They don't call Montana "Big Sky Country" for no reason. The sky there overwhelms you. It drapes over you. It runs clear across the whole landscape. There is literally nothing around you but sky—a giant midnight-colored cloak, decorated with millions upon millions of diamonds, everything held together by gravitational pull.

I raised my right arm up into the air and squinted one eye shut. I pointed to the stars above me, tracing an imaginary line from one to the next to the next. Drawing the cosmos with my fingertips. After some time, my arm slid back down to my side. I took a deep breath and slowly walked back to the tipi. Somehow, after seeing the stars, I knew my way. Somehow the darkness had up and disappeared.

This tracing of lines was familiar to me. I used to do a similar thing with my mother. Not in the sky, but directly on top of her skin.

Summer, fall, winter, or spring—it doesn't matter—my mother's body is covered in freckles. Teensy-tiny, ever-so-small, and medium-large dots decorate her body from tip to tail. When I was a little girl I used to run my fingertips along her legs and arms, tracing imaginary lines from one freckle to the next, connecting them in various patterns. For some reason this comforted me. It calmed me. Running the tips of my small fingers along her thighs or her forearm. She never asked me what I was doing. She never shooed me away. She never told me to stop and go play somewhere else. Perhaps it comforted her as well. This was her language after all, a silent and demonstrative love. A knowing that someone was interested in connecting the dots of her. The feeling of someone as they gently pulled the stitching through.

"And then this one goes to that one, and that one goes to this one," I would whisper quietly as I drew a picture in the galaxy that was right there in front of me, right on my mother's body, just resting on the surface of her skin.

My mother has always been my sky. My stars. My moon. My sun. Without me knowing it, I'd been peering into her for years trying to connect the dots. This apprenticeship, this translation had been taking place since my birth, perhaps prior.

My mother was an entire galaxy, hiding in plain sight. And now, it was as if she were whispering, "There are answers living inside of you too. Start scrying."

I crept back into the tent and nestled into my sleeping bag.

My mother, an entire solar system, a grand celestial body, was sound asleep across from me.

All I wanted to do in that moment was connect the rest of the dots, unlock the myth of it all, find out what the ending was, maybe glimpse a new beginning.

But I didn't. I couldn't. I just stared at her and asked a question as she slept.

"Are you scared?" I whispered.

She didn't answer. She didn't have to.

"Am I scared?" I whispered to myself before pausing and closing my eyes.

"Yes," I breathed in response. "Yes, I'm scared."

And this, this was my new beginning. A letting alone of her answers, a quiet, groping quest for my own. However shaky, this reach, this extension of my arms and hands into the darkness felt familiar somehow, almost instinctual.

When I woke up the next morning, I immediately felt the Tetons calling. A handful of years prior I had skied in the area, just outside of Jackson Hole, Wyoming, and I remembered thinking how nice it would be to explore the national park in the summer. This is how I decided to take my mother south. Although our exact route was still unknown, our destination was clear—my mother and I were headed to Grand Teton National Park.

We both had hot showers in the facilities provided, and after eating breakfast and rolling up our sleeping bags, we thanked Angelika and Darrell for their hospitality. By nine o'clock we were on the road with clean underarms and freshly washed hair. I wasn't sure how far we would get, but the day felt promising.

We drove on a long, straight stretch of road for the first hour or two. It was boring but blissfully easy driving. And then we hit the mountains—the Sawtooths, the Elkhorns, the Big Belt Mountains, and eventually, by way of a circuitous route, the Tobacco Root Mountains and the Bitterroot Range. Fold after fold of earth, wrinkle after wrinkle of rock that help make up a portion of the great Rocky Mountains.

In the years prior to this trip, I had spent a lot of time in the mountains, mostly on skis—hours, and days, and weeks if not years of my life wandering up and skiing straight down them. In that time, I came to develop a lot of respect for mountains, singular peaks and whole ranges. In a way, I had become jealous of them, of the way they just were. The way they can just stand there and quietly endure. The way they let life come in and carve something out of them astounded me. Up until a few years prior my whole life had been an attempt at the opposite—me in some attempt to control. For surely, I was not the thing to be carved, but the carver itself.

I glanced at my mother in the passenger seat of the car. A woman cast by the wind and rain, sleet and snow; shaped by the tectonic plates beneath her.

She looked back at me and smiled before holding up a map for me to see.

"Where are we on this?" she asked.

"I don't know, Mom," I said. "But next time we stop, I'll take a look."

"Okay," she said, before continuing on with a quiet examination of the map.

At the beginning of our trip my mother had spotted a few pages of maps at the back of our guidebook. She immediately commented on how handy they would be. I agreed with her, all the while knowing we wouldn't need them. I had my phone, which came with a fully functioning GPS system.

Every time we got in the car, she asked for those maps, and I happily fulfilled her request. I figured they would be the perfect distraction—the Alzheimer's road-trip equivalent of giving a child an iPad preloaded with all of their favorite videos.

I figured wrong. The whole situation made me feel like I was driving with Siri, only Siri kept forgetting where we were, where we were going, and what map she should be using.

Until that day, the fixation my mother had about identifying exactly where we were at any given moment hadn't mattered that much. Most of our drives had been fairly short, but three hours and 137 variations in on the question "Where are we?" had me very close to losing my temper. And then I saw it—the small orange gas tank warning light in the dash of the car had switched on.

How did I not notice that? I thought to myself.

This thought was followed quite quickly by another.

Where are we? I wondered.

Because even though I had answered that question close to two hundred times already, I really did need to know.

I couldn't ask my mom to Google the next town or to figure out where the closest gas station was without confusing the heck out of her and simultaneously losing my shit. So I just brushed it all aside and figured we were where we were and there was bound to be a gas station just around the bend.

Again, I figured wrong.

There was not a gas station just around the bend, and there was not a gas station just around the bend of that bend. About twenty-five miles after the light had come on, in the midst of the very meandering route we had taken, we were still who knows how far from a gas station.

This was when I started to panic. I continued driving, my body rooted in place while my mind scattered into the future, imagining various scenarios to come.

If we ran out of gas, if I had to pull the car over on the side of the road, do I bring my mother with me or do I leave her in the car? If I left her, would she stay there? Would she wait, or would she wander off? Okay, so I bring her . . . but how long would we be walking in the cold, on a cold road, toward a cold town, in the middle of cold, cold nowhere? Where is her hat? How much water do we have? What kind of shoes does she have on?

I scanned my brain trying to remember what town we had most recently passed, and how far back it had been.

Good God, that was a long way back, I thought to myself. *At least forty miles . . . way too late to turn back. Why didn't I just fill up when we left Browning?!*

My mind flashed to something my friend Sarah had recently sent me—a text with a photo of some contraption designed to squeeze toothpaste out of its tube, every ounce of it.

"You need this," she wrote in her text.

It's an ongoing joke between me and anyone who knows me. I like finishing things. I like to see tubes and jars and containers completely empty before I fill them again or open a new one. It's a mild obsession. Something about it brings me joy. But this time, it was about to shoot me in the foot, and potentially take out my dear, sweet mother as well—death by freezing on the long walk to a gas station far, far away.

My panic moved like a current of electricity through the car. It moved straight out my arms and into the air before landing squarely in front of my mother. She placed the map in her lap.

"What's wrong?" she asked abruptly.

"Nothing," I lied, biting the inside of my lip.

A minute or two went by.

"What's wrong?" she asked again.

All of the truth, I said to myself.

"Well," I said, my voice short and tight. "We're *really* close to running out of gas."

"How close?" she asked, while glancing at the map she had just put down.

I didn't respond.

We passed a sign. It did not have a gas icon on it, nor did it read GAS—10 MILES.

We passed another sign. Nothing.

"Oh my fuck," I said aloud.

My panic had escalated, and my mother's raised up to match. She picked the map up from her lap and had what she thought was an ah-ha.

"Oh!" she said, holding it up in the air. "I'll look on the map!"

And then she paused.

"But . . . I've lost where we were. Where are we?"

Something inside of me exploded.

"I don't know where we are!" I shouted.

I felt my mother flinch. Her whole little body—it was like watching a tiny bird startling in the seat beside me.

"Mom," I said. "I'm sorry. I'm so sorry. It's just that the map isn't going to help us right now."

"What do you mean it won't help us?" she asked. "How will we know where we're going?"

She had forgotten about the gas. I held my breath. In that moment, my frustration would not allow a reply.

She stared at me for a bit longer.

"I'd like to help," she said, softly, tentatively. "But if I don't know where we are on the map, I can't help. I won't be able to tell you which direction to go."

I shrank down in my seat, and let out a large sigh. I forgot about the gas.

My mother didn't have a desperate need to know exactly where she was at any given moment. She was just trying to help me. My mom didn't care where she was on the map, she cared about being kind and supportive. She wasn't trying to keep track of anything for the sake of keeping track. She was trying to make sure we didn't get lost.

My mother was trying to make sure I didn't get lost.

I flashed back to all the family road trips we had taken growing up. The two-tone Volkswagen van. My mother's car, the car that all the kids fit into, the best option for field trips, playdate pickups, and soccer games. And although I know she drove it most of the time, I can't pull up a single memory of what she looked like behind the wheel. All I can see is my dad driving out of town as we headed off for a weekend or short family vacation, his right hand on the gearshift, my mom in the front passenger seat beside him, her hands managing the creases of an oversized, foldout map. All I can see is her finger tracing our route up and out of the valleys and on into the mountains beyond.

My mother held the map for all of us. My mother was trying to make sure we didn't get lost.

In that moment, I realized that she too had things to let go of.

I looked up and saw a sign for a small town. I didn't see a gas icon, but I knew I had to pull in regardless. I had to ask someone for help. My mother and I needed some help.

The town itself was ridiculously small, a speck of a place, really. There was one road, a handful of houses with beat-up wood-post fences, and a fish tackle / trading post–type shop with an old Wild West frontage. Beside the shop, I noticed an empty lot with, miraculously, a single gas pump just sort of plunked down on the asphalt.

I parked the car beside it and told my mom I'd be right back. Once out of the car, I realized that the pump might not actually be a pump. It was beyond dated, like so dated it could have been installed sometime around the turn of the century, the turn prior to the one we just had. There was a chance it was decorative, a relic from days of yore, something kerosene once came out of.

And even if it did work, it did not look like the kind of

thing I would be able to operate without help. On top of that, there was no one around to pay.

I waved to my mom, and even though things were not going that well, I gave her the thumbs-up. She gave one in return from the car.

I made my way over to the tackle shop and walked in.

There was a man dressed in camouflage clothing standing behind the desk. He did not greet me.

"Hi," I said, hesitantly.

He still did not greet me.

"Um . . . I was wondering . . . do you know about the gas pump next door?"

He said nothing.

"You see, my mother and I are really close to running out of gas, and I sure could use some help."

The man stared at me blankly, pushed his sleeves up his arms, and then turned to look out the window behind him.

He could see the pump and the car from where he stood.

"Fuckin'—" he said, mumbling a name I could not make out. "Sorry 'bout that," he added. "He's s'pposed to be out there. And he's never out there."

"Oh," I said. "Okay. Well, is it possible to, like, call him or something?"

"No," he said bluntly. "But I'll tell ya what. You can pay me, I'll help ya out, and then I'll pay 'im if he ever comes back. Or maybe I won't, but you can leave that to me."

"Okay," I said. "Sounds like a plan."

"How much d'ya want?" he asked, as he started in on ringing up a charge for me.

"As much as I can get," I said. "Maybe fifty bucks."

The man laughed.

"Oh, he's gonna be pissed to have missed a sale like that," he said. "Now, come on and I'll show ya how this old thing works."

We walked out of the shop and over to the car. I waved again to my mom, and she waved back.

"That yer mom?" asked the man, as he started filling the tank for me.

"Yep," I said.

"Looks like a nice lady."

"She is," I said. "She's a really nice lady."

When the tank was full, I thanked him for his help and hopped back in the car.

"Everything okay?" asked my mom.

"Yep," I said, as I started the car and pulled back out onto the road. "That was a close call but we're fine."

But my mom wasn't listening for my response. She was looking down at her lap.

"I was wondering," she said, as she picked up the map. "Where are we, exactly?"

I looked out the window and saw a sign.

"We're in Wisdom, Mom. Wisdom, Montana. Population ninety-eight."

"And where is that on this ma—"

"You know, Mom, we don't have a map of this area," I lied. "But you know what you can do to be helpful? You can high-five me every time you see a red car."

"That will be helpful?" she asked.

"Super helpful," I said.

"Okay. If you're sure."

"I'm sure, Mom. A high five for every red car, and why don't we tuck that map away. It's not for this area."

About two hours later I caught my mom looking out the window of the car. Her face was relaxed and blissful. We were somewhere in Idaho, and we had already high-fived about seventeen times. Everything around us was green, a chlorophyll carpet of fresh spring, just now emerging from the ground.

I pulled the car over so I could get out and take a photo, and as I did, my mom turned to me.

"I like it when you do that," she said.

"Do what?" I asked.

"Drive over those things."

She was referring to the rumble strips on the side of the road.

"Why's that?" I asked, with a laugh.

She smiled at me sheepishly.

"They tickle my bum," she said, before bursting into laughter.

We drove close to 500 miles that day before landing in Idaho Falls just before dark. I didn't have it in me to search for a place to camp, so we grabbed a hotel room in town. After that many nights on the road it felt strange, almost disorienting, to be so surrounded by people and concrete, to tuck ourselves into beds with clean, white sheets.

When we woke up the next morning, we took a long walk along the greenbelt that hugs the Snake River. Up one side of town and down the other before arriving back where we'd started.

Sometimes it's hard to know if you're walking in circles or if you're somehow spiraling upward, repeating various points on your journey in some sort of grand ascension. Sometimes it's hard to know if you're moving away from or toward a place called wisdom. There's not a map in the world that will tell you the answer.

Although my feet were planted on a large expanse of pavement, I felt wobbly and disconnected. I wanted to be back in the dirt. I hadn't realized how steady it had made me feel, being so close to the earth for that many days in a row. How grounded I was when surrounded by all those forests and mountains and clear alpine lakes. How nurturing it had felt to be tucked inside a vast expanse of darkness. A womb. A safe place for the re-creation of self.

16

The Movement of Stone

*Wholeness is not achieved by cutting off a
portion of one's being, but by integration of
the contraries.*

—CARL JUNG

We got in the car that afternoon and drove across the Idaho–
Wyoming state line, and then up and over the Teton Pass. We
cruised into the valley that surrounds the town of Jackson,
and then onto a road that runs beside a sweeping expanse of
land—the National Elk Refuge, one of the largest of its kind
on earth. About forty miles north of that, we pulled up to the
kiosk of a camping area on the shores of Jackson Lake. I already felt more sure-footed.

We paid a small fee and received a site number as well as
some maps before driving into the grounds. It was official. We
were in Grand Teton National Park.

As soon as I pulled the car into our plot, my mom announced that she had to go pee.

"Good timing," I said, as I reached for the campsite map that was sitting on the dash. It looked as though our site was relatively close to the women's toilets—behind us, and one site over. I got out of the car and walked to the back edge of our site. I could see the entrance from where I stood.

"Do you see it there, Mom?" I asked, pointing toward the small building. "That's the washroom. The toilets are in there."

"Okay," she said quietly, not moving from where she stood.

"Are you okay to go on your own?" I added.

"You don't have to go too?" she asked. This was a passive way of her saying she would feel better if I went with her. But I was tired, it was going to be dark soon, and I wanted to get dinner going.

"No," I said. "I don't have to go. I was going to start making dinner."

"Oh," she said.

"Do you want me to come with you?" I asked.

At this point in my mom's progression I wasn't worried about anything other than her figuring out how to flush if the toilet had a nontraditional lever and/or getting a bit turned around on the way out. But there really was no way for her to get lost. All I had to do was keep my eye on the main door and call her back to the site if I saw she was confused. We were only a few steps away.

"I can go on my own," she said, before pointing over to the washrooms. "It's just right there, right?"

"Yep. Just over there," I confirmed. "And I'm right here. I'll keep my eye on the door."

I watched my mom walk out of the bathrooms five minutes later, happy as a clam. She peeked around, saw me waving, and then walked straight back to help me set up.

Not even six months later, there's no way I would have done anything other than walk with her and wait for her outside of the building. A year after that I would be in the building, by the sinks, making sure she remembered to wash her hands. Another stretch of months would go by and I would be outside the stall, answering questions and reminding her to throw the toilet paper into the toilet (as opposed to folding the soiled scraps and tucking them into her pocket or her purse). Soon enough she would forget about toilet paper altogether and I would help her scrub her fouled hands. After that I would rub her back, ask her to lean forward, and take care of the entire process on her behalf. This is the progression of Alzheimer's. It's not just someone who gets turned around on the way back from the bathrooms or is forgetful about names and places and faces. It is a slow and steady scraping away of one's dignity. It is the exposure of self at the most vulnerable and intimate level.

The clouds arrived as soon as we had eaten the last bite of our dinner. A thick, navy cloak swung swiftly across the sky.

"We should set up the tent," I said to my mom. "I think it's going to rain."

"The tent?" she asked. "What tent? Are we sleeping here?"

The number of things my mother doesn't know grows larger every day. It feels to me like she is wandering aimlessly from here to there. Or maybe it's me. Maybe the truth of it is that I feel like I'm wandering aimlessly from here to there.

We worked quickly. Or more accurately, I worked quickly while simultaneously answering her questions about what we were doing, what this pole thingy was, where the zipper zipped, and again . . . what we were doing.

As I pounded the last stake into the ground, I felt a few drops of rain hit the back of my neck.

"Okay! Looks good," I said, before hustling toward the car. "Come on, Mom . . . it's starting to rain."

We hopped inside the car and spent a few hours there to avoid the damp. I popped a headlamp on top of my mother's beanie, and she started in on coloring a plant-based mandala. I watched her for a moment or two, and I felt myself getting agitated.

I heard my aunt's voice in my head: *She just sat there and painted, colored. Every day for a year.*

I felt something, some energy, snake its way up my thighs, leaving them feeling vacant, cold, and a little bit numb. The energy moved into my stomach; the quivering of it made me feel like I was going to be sick.

I took a deep breath and I reached for my phone, wishing to be distracted. But it was dead.

Okay, I thought to myself. *Okay.*

I put the phone down on the dash of the car and placed my hands in my lap. And then, because I wasn't sure what to do, I fidgeted. I twiddled my fingers together for a while, before moving them to the tops of my thighs, where they began to gently tap.

Tap, tap, tap.

I looked at the rain coming down on the windshield, and then I paused for a moment to listen.

Tap, tap, tap.

I rubbed my hands along the tops of my legs, pressing down rather firmly, and I let out a large exhale. As I did, I heard the rain come down even harder. It bore down on the windshield and the roof of the car. It pummeled the ground all around us. This was sky in the midst of release. Something had built up inside of it, and it was time to let that thing go. And it would use no words to do it, just energy in motion and a little bit of sound.

I sat there, heeding the lesson being offered by the sky. I rubbed my legs until they didn't feel so numb. I let my discomfort roll in waves through my stomach and chest. I shook my arms and hands, flicking anger and frustration from my fingertips, as opposed to my essence. I felt heat in my chest and my throat. I took a deep breath in, and when I let it out, it came with a sound, a peal of thunder from somewhere inside of me.

My mother looked up from her mandala, a questioning look in her eyes. I looked back at her and let lightning flicker from mine. Very slowly, she nodded her head, just once, before going back to her coloring.

What was that? I wondered. *Was that approval? Does she know what I'm doing, because I don't.*

This made me laugh a little, and as I did, I felt the torrents slow, both internally and externally. The deluge of rain turned into drizzle. My body felt relaxed, but awake, and a little bit tingly. A few more moments passed, and when the rain became nothing more than a fine mist, I moved my mother and me from the car to the tent. Once there, I handed my mom her pajamas and instructed her on how to get in them before helping her pull her sleeping bag up around her shoulders.

"It's so cozy in here," she said before falling quickly asleep. Although we still had a handful of nights left to go, I was starting to feel like I would miss my mother's nightly comments about the coziness of our tent. Nothing seemed to make her happier, more relaxed than climbing into her fluffy down bed.

I slid into my sleeping bag, and as I dozed off, I could hear water trickling from the top of our rain fly, to where it was absorbed by the earth below.

My third bear dream came that night.

I dreamt that my mother and I were sitting in the car, just as we had been a few hours prior. Only this time, instead of watching the rain, we were watching two bears. This dream was less frightening, less shocking than the two that had come prior. It was just a couple of curious bears sniffing around the car. I watched as they grabbed the windshield wipers off the front of the car and started chewing on the rubber of them, before moving to the seals on each of the doors. Both my mother and I sat wide-eyed, staring at the animals. There was an urge to start the car and drive away, but I knew it would hurt them, so we just sat there and watched as they continued to nibble away.

"They're hungry," said my mother in the dream. "They must have just woken up from their sleep."

I nodded in casual agreement.

Three, I thought the next morning. *Three bear dreams.*

I didn't know what to make of the dream, nor the two that had come prior, but as a collection I knew this trilogy of Jungian storytelling had to have some significance. So I did what every person does with the things we know we should keep, even when we're unsure of their use. I snapped a rubber band around all three dreams and placed them in the junk drawer of my brain, and then moved on to make breakfast and a big cup of coffee.

"Let's eat by the lake," I said to my mom, the drawer firmly closed in my brain.

"What lake?" she asked, as she scanned the area around us. "There's no lake here."

"Follow me," I said, while handing her a mug of steaming oatmeal and nodding toward a small trailhead across the way.

The two of us walked down the path toward the water, and as we turned the corner I heard my mom let out a small gasp.

It was her first time seeing the Grand Tetons, and "seeing" is not quite the right word. You don't "see" the Tetons, you take them in. You behold them. You wonder about the number of clouds they've sliced in half. You muse about how the jawline of a giant crocodile rose up and out of the earth. You are filled with awe, followed, almost immediately, by question after question after question.

At the very same time, when you look at their peaks—Grand Teton, Mount Owen, Teewinot, and beyond, a conspiracy of slate-shaped ravens soaring through the sky—you lay each and every one of those questions to the ground. You do this because when you're standing in front of the Tetons, you're surrounded by something bigger than you. It's inarguable. In one fell swoop,

you see the chasm between everything you know and everything you never will and never have to. In one fell swoop, you
understand God. And nothing seems to matter when you're toe
to toe with mountains like that.

I watched my mother as she locked eyes with those mountains, and although I'll never know exactly what she was thinking in that moment, what I saw and what I felt were distinctly
clear to me. A knowing flooded into my flesh. I suddenly felt like
a small child again, watching my mother in admiration. Watching her know how to do something I hadn't a clue how to do.

How to tie a shoe. How to make those birthday cakes with
icing smooth as butter. How to get the dog to sit or make a person feel better with a glass of ginger ale. How to fold a fitted
sheet, or how to have a wordless conversation with a chain link
of mountains. The feeling of amazement, of delirious reverie,
of knowing for sure when something is bigger than you—it
all came pouring back in, it soaked me, it moved through my
bones and into my marrow, the softest tissue of me.

A conversation was occurring. Information was being exchanged. I couldn't help but feel as though my mother and
those mountains were talking about making way, about allowing something to shape you—from the surface and far
below—about the cycles of death and rebirth. They saw one
another. It was a clear recognition, a dropping away of the
body, a dismissal of what we might call knowledge, a forgetting of it all so as to remember everything that ever was.

There is a type of meditation called Zuòwàng. It comes from
the Taoist tradition and translates roughly to "sitting and forgetting." The idea being that one sits and works to forget, to let go

of ego, identity, knowledge, and various mental constructs so as to slip into oneness with the world. The meditation encourages a person to "lose their mind" so as to feel, and become part of, the only thing believed to be real—otherwise known as the dao, the underlying current of energy, of mystical oneness.

My mother was sitting and forgetting. My mother was searching for enlightenment. She was spiraling in ascension. She was staring at what I saw as immovable, and yet somehow, she seemed to be watching it move. This told me everything I ever needed to know.

My dear friend Maia Toll sent me an email some time ago. In it she wrote:

So a plant that could survive in the desert, for instance, a plant that learned to hold its moisture despite the dry heat, was seen to have the medicine of water. This became the gift it could give us.

As soon as I read her email, I understood in my core what she meant.

So a woman who could survive in between a rock and the secrecy of a hard place, I thought to myself, *was seen to have the medicine of mountains, including how they move. And a child who could survive the silence of that world was seen to have the medicine of words, of the stories that wrap right around us.*

My mother gave me many things. And I didn't understand why conversation had not been one of those things. I didn't see it until that moment in Grand Teton, until I watched my mother's eyes flicker at the movement of stone. A conversation was taking place that I couldn't hear or understand. It was in a wordless language I did not know.

Every time my mother chose to be silent, to not fill the world around me with her words, she had given me a gift—space, a dazzling expanse for me to fill and fill again with my stories.

Every time my mother chose not to explain things, not to tell me all of her truth, she had been offering me something—a hollow for me to explore my truths as opposed to the ones that belonged to her.

Every time she held her tongue had been a sacrifice in my name. In a world that contained few of her words, I would have to use my senses; I would have to develop the kind of observation required to navigate the entirety of the world around me.

When my mother moved in two different directions at once, she had given me a gift—a lesson that I was never alone, that regardless of what I surrounded myself with in the external world, my internal world could provide me with an intimacy that few will ever know.

My mother, of course, knew all of this in advance. Because my mother was bigger than me. She was the one who'd come first.

Later that afternoon, my mother and I went on a guided hike. The ranger who led it offered us a bounty of information. Fact after geological fact, information about the events that carved out the cliffs and canyons, the metamorphic collisions that created the mountains soaring above us. We were told the names of the various types of dry grass and brush, as well as the differentiations between limber, lodgepole, and whitebark pine. We stopped here and there so she could point out the just-now-blooming Indian paintbrush, phlox, and cinquefoil.

I knew my mom wouldn't and couldn't take in much of the information provided. Her brain was too similar to the soil around us, what the ranger described as rather porous and rocky. Regardless, she seemed to be taking something in. Her hands turning this way or that, palms open to the warm breeze floating by. Her face raised also to the wind, so as to let the pollen brush by, painting her cheeks with a fine yellow blush as it went. Her posture shifting, pulling taller as she heard grunts coming from a scoop of nearby white pelicans. Her fingers moving across the markings we saw on a tree.

"Likely left over from last season," said the ranger. "A buck rubbing a bit of that fuzz off their antlers."

I wonder sometimes about the limits of science. I worry about our use of it as the singular lens with which to connect to the world around us, the way we surround ourselves with information, like it's a blanket that will keep us warm when the world falls apart.

I've always thought of science as a doorway into the questions of nature, as an entryway into Mother Nature's many mysteries. But I couldn't help but feel there was a larger story underneath the facts and figures we were told that day. Like something had been buried in the sediment somewhere, and that our way of communicating in Latin terminology wasn't big enough to hold it. Like there is not enough space in our

mouths to speak the language of Mother Nature, to understand what it is the earth has to say. We have to use more of
ourselves, more than our brains, more than just the statistics
and the name of the genus rolling rotely off the tip of our
tongues. Science is too new a language to contain the depths
of Mother Nature, too narrow to fit the breadth of this place.
It might be the doorway, but it is not the whole house.

I watched my mother as she stood, her feet on billion-year-
old glacial till. Every subtle movement in her body told me
she knew an older language, or at the very least, that she had
a handful of primordial words. She was leaving her brain behind so as to sink into the intelligence inside her body.

The hike came to an end, and the ranger went back to the
station. The other hikers dispersed, like ants hurrying down
this pathway and that. But my mother and I stood there for a
while longer. Side by side on the gravel path. I took her hand
in mine. I could feel my pulse beating softly against the palm
of her hand, or was that her pulse against the palm of mine? I
dropped my shoulders. I stood more softly, attempting to feel
into whose heartbeat was whose.

I heard a story once about wolves, something about how the
alpha wolves are identified, about how a pack chooses which wolf
to follow. I thought it would be about their ferocity, their ability
to track and hunt prey, but I was wrong. It's about their heart
rate. I don't know if it's true or not, but apparently the leaders
of the pack always have the steadiest rhythm. A low, humming
beat—almost silent, barely detectable—that draws the others in,
making all the wolves feel calm.

My mother is the calmest wolf. Her love is an unhurried

heartbeat. Growing up, I felt it through the palms of her hands as they held my cheeks, rubbed my back, petted my head—a sonar that pulsed steadily onward. My mother's love is an aortic repetition; it was the number of times she told me she loved me without having to make a single sound.

My wisdom was that I knew it, and that I'd known it all along; the number of times I understood what she was saying, even in the absence of words.

I too spoke this language. We all do. It resides somewhere inside of us. All we have to do is learn to dredge it up, to trust that there are silent and invisible tendrils of energy laden with truths that all of us can lean into. All we have to do is not forget it in the first place.

17

Stardust

To the ancients, bears symbolized
resurrection . . . a profound metaphor for our
lives, for return and increase coming from
something that seemed deadened.

—CLARISSA PINKOLA ESTÉS

We spent the next afternoon on horseback, before returning to the lake. I read and my mother colored until twilight
arrived—sweet-tempered twilight, asking us to watch as the
sun called everything home. A gradual shifting of colors.
Light pulled gently back up the mountain faces. And then at
last—*woosh*—a candle blown out, the hushed sound of dusk's
arrival.

What a beautiful thing it is to watch light. The line of it in
the morning, eager and unaware as it casts itself out into the
day. Soaked in the yellow buzz of youth, seemingly unfazed by
how or when it will return to its roots, perhaps even unaware

that it will. And the boldness of light at midday. How stunning. How laughable. It's wide-eyed belief that, surely, from this height no shadow could exist. And then, light's innocent waning. The discovery that there is more to the world than its illumination. And finally, its retreat. Its transformation—a steady silhouette walking all the way home as everything around it begins to fade.

I thought I knew our pattern, the dance my mother and I had done. But in the timeline of our lives, I had only watched until midday, or perhaps an hour or so after to the golden afternoon. What a glorious thing it is to be enveloped by the sun, and then to move together toward dusk. To pull away from the world, holding one another in the darkness, knowing with all of your heart that a new day will come even when you can't yet see it, even when all you can feel is the cold.

"Come on, Mom," I said, as the light dimmed around us. "Let's go make a fire."

We picked up our chairs, walked back up the trail to the campsite, and started in on the paper and kindling. It was our last night in the Tetons.

I didn't have a lot of experience chopping wood or preparing campfires, but throughout the journey with my mom, and in every fire I've lit since, I've noticed a ceremonial feeling. The dimming light—bodies slipping into silhouette, and then finally dark and voluminous shadows. The elemental sounds, and the scent of fresh birch, or perhaps cedar or ash. The way you wake in the morning with remnants of smoke on your hair.

When I struck the match that night, it felt like a summoning

208 II Everything Left to Remember

of sorts. All of the elements of magic were there. The red stripe on the side of the matchbox, made with the same minerals as are found in our teeth and our bones. The snapping sound as the match caught flame. The smell of metal and sulfur. The wood crackling, transforming itself into flame. It was an invocation, I'm sure of it, to whom or for what I didn't know.

"So warm," said my mom, as she moved a little closer to the fire.

We sat in silence for most of the night. Mesmerized, hypnotized, by the dancing light of the flames.

I don't know how much time passed, but at some point I heard my mother's voice.

"Are you tired?" she asked.

I knew this was her way of saying she wanted to go to sleep, so I ducked into the tent and grabbed her pajamas.

"Let's get you into your pj's by the fire," I said. "It's so warm over here."

As my mom got changed, I prepped her toothbrush.

"Here," I said, as I placed it in her hand. "When you're done with your teeth, why don't you climb into bed?"

"Where's bed?" she asked.

"It's in the tent. Just over here," I added.

"Here?" she asked, pointing at the tent. "Inside of this?"

I walked over and unzipped the rain fly, as well as the door of the tent.

"Yep, right in here."

"Oh, right," she said, as she climbed in. "I thought so."

She looked back at me.

"Are you coming?" she asked, as she snuggled down into her sleeping bag.

"Soon," I said. "I just have to make sure the fire is out."

I re-zipped the mesh door and then paused to look at her. She looked back.

"Thank you," she said sleepily. "This is so nice."

"You're welcome, Mom," I said, holding her gaze until she closed her eyes.

Once she was settled, I walked over to the picnic table at the edge of the campsite, grabbed our cooking pot, and filled it with some water. I made my way back to the dwindling fire, used a stick to push the remaining logs away from one another, and then I slowly poured water over the top of it all. The wood hissed. Clouds of smoke puffed into the air as the fire extinguished. The light went dark, and as it did, I stirred the ashes to make sure nothing was still burning.

With the pot still in my hand, I took a deep breath, and I looked up to the night sky. We weren't in Montana anymore, but the sky here in Wyoming seemed just as large and equally filled with starlight. Cosmic stories unfolding by way of sparkling light, the backdrop of eternity.

I saw the Big Dipper first. Three stars for the handle, and four for the bowl. I stretched my eyes out from there and landed on the Little Dipper, another ladle and bowl made with Polaris, the North Star, and six other twinkling lights.

"Ursa Major," I said quietly, whispering to the smoke and the sky. "Ursa Major and Minor."

At the time I didn't know what those Latin words meant,

nor the Greek myth that came with them. It was something I came to learn a handful of years later—and when I did, when I saw the translation, I gasped.

> Ursa Major and Ursa Minor—prominent in the northern sky in the months of May and June— otherwise known as Greater Bear and Lesser Bear.

Greater Bear and Lesser Bear. Greater Bear and Lesser Bear. Two women rocking back and forth in a galaxy made of salt water and stars.

I clicked through a handful of links until I landed on the myth of the bears. As the story goes, Zeus, the Olympian god of the sky and thunder, was having an affair with a beautiful woman named Callisto. The pair were together one day in the forest when they heard the voice of Zeus' wife. In a panic, and not wanting to be caught, Zeus turned Callisto into a bear.

"Don't worry," he said. "I'll turn you right back as soon as she's gone."

Only Zeus' wife didn't go. She told Zeus he was needed in Olympus immediately. There was only one option—just before leaving, Zeus instructed Callisto to wait in the forest. He promised he would return the next morning to reverse the spell.

Zeus and his wife promptly left. And the bear . . . the bear stood alone in the wilderness.

Shortly after, a hunter came by, spotted the bear, and immediately brought forth an arrow. The hunter took the bear down in a single lethal shot, but as the bear was dying, it turned back into Callisto. The hunter screamed twice in terror. First, because he was watching a bear turn into a woman. Second, because the hunter was Callisto's own child.

The hunter had shot his own mother.

Realizing what had just happened, the pair began to wail. They wailed with such force that their screams could be heard from Olympus. Zeus' ears filled with the sound of great sorrow. He ran back to the forest, and upon seeing the tragedy before him, he fell to his knees. The god of the sky and thunder knew only one thing to do—he turned both Callisto and the hunter into stars, making them two of the biggest constellations in the sky. Big Bear and Little Bear, the child who shot its own mother.

My brain flickered back and forth, back and forth—a crackling filament just about to pop. I saw my mother's freckles, the lines I used to trace on her arms and her legs. I yanked the junk drawer inside of my brain wide open and frantically searched for that trio of dreams, flipping through them one by one—my mother and I shape-shifting into bears, her screaming at me, me about to pounce, and then the two of us quietly watching the pair of hungry bears. And then again, like a top, my mind whirled to the image of me standing beside the tipi, arm stretched out, tracing the stars in the dark of the night.

I thought of all of the times I made my mother smaller. All of the ways society—the world around me, the gods of the sky and thunder—encouraged me to do so. All of the ways I had taken aim and shot her down. Every time I rolled my eyes before turning to my friends. "Please don't let me turn into my mother," I'd say, my tongue coated in sarcasm.

Sarcasm—a word whose Latin root means "to tear flesh."

I could see it so clearly now—the false idols, how I had projected the masculine high up in the sky, me ebbing ever outward in some mad attempt to reach it. How I bought into the lie that women and mothers were on the lesser-than side of life's long and complex comparisons. How I had been encouraged to take aim at the women around me. I could see the feminine lying facedown on the ground. I could feel the vibration of the quivering bow still moving through my arms.

My anger at the world around me, my confusion about my own worth, about being a woman in a society that glorifies the masculine, led me to shooting down my own mother. Little did I know that part of me would be lying on the ground right beside her.

My mother had been a convenient target for my rage, but it was never her I was mad at. My fury had always been about the expectation I had been handed at birth, the presumption that I live happily ever after in a society that actively denies and devalues the very essence of my being. Never once had I questioned who had placed the bow and arrow in my hands.

In that moment, I heard an echo of my mother's voice: *It never occurred to me.*

Is that what she'd said?

I didn't know this was where the journey with my mother would take me. If you had asked, I would have said that the trip we took was my way of coming to terms with the loss of her, that this was some long, excruciating walk to the burial grounds. But this was about resurrection. This was all fragments, the lost pieces, the language of our wild selves, returned to us. This was my mother and I, reclaimed and fully re-membered. This was, as Nor Hall once wrote, "a remembering . . . a putting back together of the mother-daughter body."

This was about letting the bears, the ones who had been silently raging inside of us, out into the wild, so as to let our own savage nature come flooding back into us, back into where it belonged.

This was a grand lesson passed down to me by two immeasurable women, my mother and Mother Nature—and by Alzheimer's too. It was a lesson in surrender. Surrendering the ego of the bright young maiden, so as to take in the awe-inspiring immensity of mother. A full surrender to see if once and for all I can survive, not in the wilderness that lives outside of me, but in the one that resides on the inside. To see if I can love all of myself as these two women loved me—fiercely, fully, freely.

My mother named me Stephanie, an ancient Greek name meaning "crown." My mother's name is of Irish origin—translating roughly to "heavenly." Together we make a heavenly crown.

My mother is part woman and part bear in the sky. She is what the Taoists call ch'i, the magnetic and vital life force that flows between the North Star and the Big Dipper. She is starlight in motion. She is a cosmos of jewels, jewels I will wear until I am ready to join her. Until one day, I too am made luminescent.

What a beautiful thing it is to watch the stars, knowing they reside somewhere inside of you, certain that the single most important job you have is to become more and more of them until—poof—you've arranged yourself inside the lineage, an ancestral constellation.

A billion years, as astronomer Jill Tarter would say, of wandering stardust.

When I slipped into the tent that night, my body felt like honey. I slept soundly all through the night. It was our last night of camping on this trip, and very likely our last time camping together at all. I surrendered. All I had to do was lie there, sleeping next to my mother.

18

My Mother Tongue

To put your hands in a river is to feel the
chords that bind the earth together.

—BARRY LOPEZ

The alarm on my phone went off around 5:45 in the morning.
I opened my eyes, reached for the phone, and turned off the
alarm. It was still dark, deliciously so.

"Mom," I whispered. "It's time to get up."

I hated to disturb her sleep, but I had made plans for our
day.

She mumbled something in half confirmation.

I grabbed the headlamp I kept in the upper pocket of the
tent, flicked it on, and began fumbling around for my sports
bra, undies, and socks.

"Mom," I whispered again. "We have to wake up now."

I watched as she blinked her eyes open, registering whose

voice she was hearing, searching for information on where she was.

"It's morning?" she asked.

"Yep," I said quietly. "It's morning and we have to wake up."

She pulled her arm out of her sleeping bag and pushed the sleeve of her left wrist up. She peered down at her watch.

"I can't see," she said. "What time is it?"

"It's early," I said. "But we have something fun to do today. Up we get."

I pushed my sleeping bag down, wriggled out of my pajamas, and got myself dressed. After that, I reached for the pile of my mother's clothes I'd set aside the night prior.

"Here, Mom," I said, talking gently. "Up, up, up we get."

By then she was beginning to wiggle out of her sleeping bag.

"Ooooh. It's cold," she said.

"Put these on quick," I said, handing her the warmest clothes we'd packed. "I'm gonna go get us ready."

I put my headlamp on, unzipped the tent, and walked to the back of the car. I pulled out the stove, made a quick cup of coffee, and slapped together a few peanut butter and jelly sandwiches. Breakfast on the road.

I looked over to the tent and saw my mom slowly crawling out of it.

"Your shoes are right there," I said, pointing to the pair of running shoes I had placed just inside the rain flap.

"It's still pretty dark," she said, while tying her shoes. "Are you sure it's morning?"

"I'm sure," I confirmed. "We woke up early because we're going on a float today. A little river trip."

"Oh," she said. "Is Brian coming?"

"Nope, Dad's not here. Just you and me."

"Who's . . ." She paused to think. "Who's with the kids?"

She squinted a bit and looked around the campsite, a mixture of Alzheimer's-based confusion about where she was, combined with a thick morning grogginess.

I handed her the sandwiches.

"Will you hold these?" I asked. "We'll eat them in the car."

"Who's with the kids?" she asked again, a little more awake than before.

"Dad," I said, as I motioned for her to head to the car. "Dad's with the kids. Off we go."

"We just leave everything here?" she asked.

"Yep. We'll be back later today to pack everything up."

"Bu—"

"Mom. We'll be back," I said, cutting her off. "Seat belt, please."

We drove out of our campsite due south. The sun, although up, hadn't quite tipped over the peaks of the mountains. The light of the day was unfolding, a linen tablecloth lifted gently in the air, before settling into its place on the table. Nothing and no one around for miles.

We ate our sandwiches in silence, and I sipped on my coffee, wishing the cup would fill up again the moment it was empty. Soon enough the sun peaked and began to light the stone faces to the west of us. About thirty minutes later, we pulled into a large gravel parking lot near the southern entrance of the park.

The float was set to take place on the Snake River, the

largest tributary of the Columbia. A belt of water that rises in western Wyoming before running in a U-shape through the southern plains of Idaho.

We waited in the parking lot as a small group gathered. Everyone was silent, moving to and fro in an effort to stay warm. I looked down at my feet, and then to my mother's. Both of us were, rather oddly, standing steady.

How long have we been still? I wondered to myself.

A guide arrived shortly thereafter. He greeted us all and explained the plan for our morning. We were to pop on some life jackets, board the ten- or twelve-person raft, and then sit back and relax so as to enjoy the float downriver.

"Just a gentle glide," he said, before continuing on to tell us where he would be seated, how he would be in charge of the paddles, and how, at the end of it all, we would be shuttled back to where we began.

"If you ask me, y'all picked the best trip," said the guide. "More wildlife out on the river at dawn than there is any other time of day."

The two-hour trip started at a place called Deadman's Bar. We loaded into the boat and set off, carried slowly by the gentle flow of the water. The river itself was flanked with cottonwood and spruce forests, sagebrush plateaus up on top of the high bank. I snuggled right into my mom and put my arm around her shoulder.

"You warm enough?" I asked.

When she didn't answer, I looked into her eyes. They had a soft liquid center. She was already watching the water.

All morning long, the boat moved steadily around bars of sand and silt. We saw birds in every direction—hawks and large falcons soared at great heights up above us; great blue herons and white trumpeter swans waded in and swam through the water. And smaller birds, various types of swallow and dipper, flitted here and there—from the water to the river bank, before landing on long marshy reeds. We saw obvious evidence of beavers, but no actual beavers came out to say hello. That said, the hooved mammals made up for it. We caught glimpses of elk, deer, pronghorn, and moose as they moved through the protection of the brush along the side of the river.

Our river guide relayed many interesting facts and figures about the area, just as the ranger in Grand Teton had. But I wasn't terribly interested, for I was being flooded with remembrance, with the words of a language I knew but had forgotten how to speak.

Things were being said in that language all around us. Stories coming in on the wings of the birds, on the wind, on the river as it cut arcs through the sand on the banks. It seemed there was a whispered narrative coming in on the heartbeats of the animals walking through the brush, on the scent of pine as it warmed in the morning sun. Wisdom was pouring in on the wordlessness around us. Not by way of the technical descriptions or statistics of the area, but on the gaps in between. It came in on the spaces. It hung, like I had all my life, on the things not said.

I watched my mother catch wisdom with her body. I did

my best to do the same. Various forms of story, streams of information, were moving through the air, through the water, through an underground network of roots, and we were using our bodies in some attempt to translate it. To let all of the intelligence of the natural world brush up against us, to let it merge with our human nature.

"The goal," wrote Joseph Campbell, "is to make your heartbeat match the beat of the universe, to match your nature with nature."

It was a remembering, a letting alone of our cognition so as to have our senses flood with knowing. It was a forgetting of one's intellectual self so as to tune more deeply into the layers and nuance of who we really are. It was the act of pulling ancient knowing to the surface.

This was a language my mother and I had always spoken. It is the language of our truest belonging, our first howls of hunger, the baying in our bones before words have had a chance to arrive. It is the language of our ravenous thirst, the ache of our grief and our love.

I once heard the poet Marilyn Nelson talking about the importance of stories. "If we erase our stories, we erase our existence," she said.

As we floated down the Snake River, I thought about the wordless language, the silent discourse spoken in signs, symbols, and sensations. Patterns, textures, and vibrations. This is the language of surrender; encoded inside of it, a silent vocabulary of faith. It is the wisdom of water.

Women are the keepers of this language—held back from

traditional learning, from school and books and science, for so long we had to develop alternate ways to understand the world around us. We used our senses to catch information and our bodies to translate what was there. We developed a spirituality that was deeply interwoven with nature because we weren't permitted in the inner sanctums of our various religions. We developed a carnal knowledge, the type that is true to the Latin translation—a knowing from the flesh. This language, this is our mother tongue.

In the midst of my mother's forgetting, she was teaching me to remember this language, to use it to re-recognize the self I had long left behind. She was teaching me not to return to her, but to return to myself, so as to move toward the woman I have the chance at becoming.

I saw my path forward. All I had to do was trust that something inside of me knew how to keep walking. I had to believe that when my mind had run its course, something inside of my body held enough wisdom to guide me. And I had to have faith that this, of all things, was my birthright.

The inheritance given to me by my mother was not her story, but the ability to feel into mine. *This* was feminine knowing. This was my body understanding I had nothing more to learn and everything left to remember.

I looked over to my mother. We smiled at one another. She didn't say anything and neither did I. Words were too small for this occasion, something we both knew inside of our bones.

So instead we let the water take over, we gave in to the sensation of it carrying us from one place to the next. We trusted it would do what it has always done.

I untied us from our story, and my mother and I floated down a river made of loose strings. Transitioning. Transforming. Transmuting. We could hear our guide in the background. He talked about the life cycle of the Grand Teton watersheds, and my mother and I . . . we felt them pulsing through us.

Evaporation. Transpiration. Condensation. Precipitation. Runoff. Percolation.

Shock. Denial. Anger. Bargaining. Loneliness. Acceptance. Life. Death. Life.

Drop after drop of rain, slowly becoming the ocean itself.

I understand now why my mother loves looking at water. It's the enchantment of transmutation. It is the wordless fluidity of the feminine, fluency in the thousands of other languages available to us, the ones that course through the marrow of our bones like music moving through a bamboo reed. It's the excitement of watching something that hardly exists turn into something that is inarguably, abundantly alive. It's watching the water break right into creation. It is the mirror held up by a great and grand mother, casting back a reflection of who we are as women.

After the float, my mother and I made our way back to our campsite. From there, we packed up our things and drove north. We had the afternoon and early evening to explore before catching a very early flight out of Bozeman the next morning. This was our final leg of the journey, the last arc we would make before arriving back in the place where it all began.

Almost as soon as we hit the road, my mother turned to face me. She had a slightly panicked look in her eyes.

"What time is it?" she asked. "I think . . . oh gosh—I have to get home to the kids!"

I told her that Dad was at home with the kids.

"He is?" she asked. "They're all there?"

"Some of them are at school," I lied. "And some of them are probably having a nap. But Dad's with them."

My mother sighed.

"Oh, good," she said. "I was worried for a moment."

My mother has forgotten many things, the fact that her children are grown being one of them. Shortly after her diagnosis, and in the years that followed, her most frequent concern was the kids.

"Where are the kids?" she would ask in a panic. "Who's with the kids?"

"Oh my gosh," she would say, as she glanced at her watch. "I have to get home to the kids."

That is the one thing my mother has never let go of. Still, to this day. Her brain has yet to forfeit this fact. She may not know that she is the mother of me, but she knows, beyond a shadow of a doubt, that she is a mother. Amidst all of the forgetting, some part of her remembers this. Perhaps it was part of her contract, the fine print that the Universe, and her mother, and little bits of her soul haggled over before agreeing to drop her into the arms of my ancestors.

My mother is made of unfettered love; it is the single thread that runs through her and beyond. She is numinosity incarnate. Motherhood has been divinely imprinted over top of her soul, and it makes me wonder what, if anything, has been imprinted on mine.

19

The Path Toward Remembrance

The Achilles heel of consciousness is that we
forget. We forget what we stand for. We forget
to maintain good relations with the people
around us.

—BARRY LOPEZ

The most direct route to Bozeman took us back through Yellowstone National Park. I was happy about this, as there were a handful of sights we had missed on our first pass-through—namely, Old Faithful, as well as Grand Prismatic Spring.

My plan was to drive through the southwest section of the park to visit these two sites before heading out of the park and back to the city for an early dinner. We made it to the southern entrance by midmorning and pulled into a parking lot that was bursting with people. We circled in the car for some time before finding a spot back behind the visitor's center. After that, we simply followed the crowds—a swarm of people moving down the boardwalks.

Although not the biggest geyser in the world, as its burst of water is not the largest or tallest, Old Faithful is the most regular, hence its name. Since Yellowstone was established as a national park in 1872, there have been over one million eruptions. These days, this underground spring of boiling water blows about twenty times per day. Nearly three million people per year drive into this parking lot and walk out to the viewing platform to catch sight of Old Faithful as she sends giant bursts of water straight up into the air. On that day, my mother and I were among them—temporary devotees of the water-based volcano, the land-based whale.

"What's happening here?" she asked, as we walked toward the viewing platform that was chockablock with people.

I could see the geyser steaming in the background.

"Look, Mom," I said, as I pointed through the crowds toward the large mound of earth in front of us. "Do you see the steam?"

My mom nodded.

"I think it's about to erupt," I announced.

My mom shot me a look.

"Do we want to be here for that?!" she asked.

I laughed.

"Yes," I said. "We do. We'll be fine if we stand here. Can you see?"

She nodded again.

A few seconds later, Old Faithful erupted while cameras clicked and hundreds of people oohed and aahed.

And as soon as it was over, the throngs of people went back to their cars and drove off. Box checked.

I watched them as they dispersed. Like ants hurrying, hurrying. Hurrying where?

I felt strangely embarrassed by this behavior. Is this how we're supposed to interact with nature? Is all that's required that we drive into a crowded parking lot, run across the pavement to watch an eruption of steam for, hmmm, approximately two minutes, and then head back to the car? Is that what we grant? Two minutes to impress us with your most fantastical and then we're out—an audience with something more important to see, more boxes to check off their list. We spend more time in the souvenir shop buying T-shirts and fridge magnets.

It made me feel like we were cheating Mother Nature, like we were cheating ourselves. Like we weren't really seeing beauty as beauty, or bigness as bigness. We weren't attending to her in the same way she was attending to us.

But who was I to talk? Hadn't I done the exact same thing with my mother? Hadn't I done the exact same thing with nature? The answer was yes. My mother had an indent on her right thumb and pointer finger, the place where she's pressed down on pencil crayons. I had the same on my right middle and pointer fingers, the place where the bow had dug in, evidence of how many times I'd brought out my quiver of arrows.

Once the crowds had driven off, I turned to my mom and told her I had to use the bathroom.

"Do you need to go too?" I asked.

She didn't.

There weren't many people around, nor were there places

for her to wander, so I told her to wait for me. I left her on one of the benches in the viewing area and I dashed inside.

When I came back a few minutes later, there she was—sitting on that bench. I watched her from afar for some time. She was wearing her red zip-up sweater, and her black purse was on the bench beside her, tucked close. She was sitting tall but relaxed, and both of her feet were planted square on the ground. She just sat there facing Old Faithful. By this point, there was not a single other person around. Just my mother, and the world's most predictable geyser.

And once again, it was almost as if I could hear Old Faithful talking to my mom, whispering a lesson on the wind. I stood very still, and softly, subtly, I felt a whole world open up. I felt as though I was watching words floating on the thermals—a sort of call and response about dormancy and eruption, about what we need to carry and what we need to throw into the air, the tempests inside of us that belong in the sky. I watched as my mother soaked all of it up, ancient erudition shooting straight from the center of stone.

I took many photos that day, but the ones of my mother, alone with Old Faithful, are numinous. She was the only person out of hundreds if not thousands who stayed a while longer, who looked for something more than the show. My mother on a pew, sitting in front of the altar of everything and nothing at once.

Eventually, I took a seat beside her.

"Pretty, isn't it?" I asked, as I slipped my arm through hers. She didn't look at me. She didn't answer.

"Can we eat lunch here?" she finally asked.

"We sure can," I said. "Why don't I grab a few things from the car. We'll have a picnic."

My mother nodded, still staring at Old Faithful.

After lunch, we hopped back in the car and worked our way over to Grand Prismatic Spring, the most otherworldly part of Yellowstone.

We navigated another overflowing parking lot and began following the mass of people. I grabbed my mother's hand and led her to the start of a long, looped boardwalk. For the first few steps there was not much to see, but we were suddenly absorbed in a puff of steam.

"Here," I said to my mom, reaching for her sunglasses. "Let's put these in your purse."

Her glasses were almost completely fogged over, filled with condensation from the steam all around us.

"That's better!" she said, as I popped them into a case in her purse. "I couldn't see a thing."

"Hey, Mom," I added. "While we're here, let's put that purse strap over your head. I'd hate for anything to drop down into the water."

"What water?" she asked, as I helped her move the strap across her body.

I grabbed her hand and led her a bit further down the board-walk. After a few feet we noticed two small pools to our right. We moved to the edge and allowed people to pass as we took them both in. Each had rich, rust-colored edges and bright blue water, but the second pool was a milkier green. The signage beside us listed these as Turquoise and Opal Pool, respectively.

My mother turned to me and made a funny face.

"They look like eyes," she said, as she tilted her head to one side and added a few slow blinks for comedic impact.

I laughed.

"One of them is your eye color and the other is Granny's," I said.

She tilted her head to the other side and blinked again.

"You're right!" she added cheekily.

I put my arm around her shoulder and hugged her.

"Let's see what the other one looks like," I said, before slowly ushering us back into the file of people.

After a few minutes of shuffling we saw it. The most spectacular cauldron I had ever laid eyes on. A mesmerizing array of colors, technicolor embers in liquid form. The Eye of Horus simmering, shimmering on the surface of the earth.

My mother gasped. Something about this felt supernatural. Some highly saturated version of everything that is nature all in one glimpse, an eyeful of creation. It felt like we were standing on the cusp of a rusted chalice, like we had the opportunity to peer down into it and steal a glance of something—the answer to it all, perhaps.

A friend of mine recently returned home from a trip to Europe. She talked about visiting old ruins and taking in all of the architecture—Gothic, Renaissance, Baroque, and more. She described the buildings with awe, and then she said, "It's just so strange that we don't have that here."

"What do you mean?" I asked.

"Like why didn't the native people build things like that?" she added.

Our conversation wove around the idea of divinity from there—did permanence or impermanence make something more or less divine? What was the spiritual difference between wealth and accumulation, as opposed to reciprocity and preservation, about ownership versus kinship.

We didn't land anywhere in particular, but we both agreed that if your sacred sites were places like Yellowstone, Yosemite, and Sequoia, you probably wouldn't feel the need to build yourself an abbey.

Imagine, if you will, stumbling upon a place like Grand Prismatic Spring. Imagine being out for a walk just a few hundred years ago. Let's say you were crossing the plains. Let's say you saw steam somewhere in the horizon. Imagine getting closer. Feeling the heat. Seeing it for the first time, with no boardwalks or signs to tell you precisely what it is and how it was created.

My guess is that you would just stand there, attempting to take in the sheer impossibility of it—the miraculous earth rainbow in front of your eyes. That you would work to wrap not just your brain but your whole self around its raw and dazzling beauty. You would be transfixed. You would mutter something: "Our Mother here on earth, hallowed be thy name." You would walk home in a stupor, wondering how you were going to convince your family that you just saw evidence of God, a manifestation of her right here on earth. Wondering how you would tell them that something, somewhere out there, branded you, left a wordless mark on your soul.

Much of Yellowstone, including Grand Prismatic Spring, was, and still is, a sacred meeting place for Native American peoples. We have forgotten this. We have taken their Dome of the Rock, their Western Wall, their Sepulchre, and their St. Peter's and we have claimed them as ours. We have forgotten that we are walking on holy ground, that we are placing our feet at a narrow gate, a colorful chasm that marks the space between heaven and earth.

How is it possible to claim a place like Grand Prismatic Spring? To call it ours when clearly it has always belonged to itself?

And then I remembered the thoughts that had risen up inside of me while we were on Blackfeet land:

We do this with land. And we do this with people too.

How did we come to believe that our Mother owed her whole self to us? How did we become so convinced that all of this was ours?

We think we're bigger than she is. But she came first. And all she wants is to be seen . . . and remembered.

There is a GIF that exists somewhere on the internet. It's a time-lapse video that takes its viewer through the history of Indian land cessions in the United States. The images flip from 1784 all the way through to present-day reservation holdings. They show a recession, an all but disappearance. They show an ebb, a tide sweeping across the landscape, only ever moving in a singular diminishing direction.

One could make a very similar video to demonstrate deforestation in the United States. Or another to show how the habitats of birds, and then the birds themselves, have disappeared in a similar way, over a similar time span.

As my mother and I stood in front of those springs, the smell of sulfur wafting through the air, I realized that another video could be made. An eerily similar video using scans of my mother's brain, as well as scans from the brains of the 1,300 people who would be diagnosed with Alzheimer's in the time that it took us to get back to Vancouver.

This last video could be called a GIF of forgetting. They could all be called GIFs of forgetting.

As we stood there together, I heard the voice again. The words of it weren't quite clear, but in my stillness, letting the steam from the springs meet my face, letting mist land on the tops of my hands and bedew the small hairs on my arms, I swore I could hear it.

"You are in the midst of a mass forgetting of essence," it whispered like an aspen tree, like a snake, like the wings of a black-chinned hummingbird. "You are forgetting yourself and me with it."

I reached for my mother's hand.

Is that what we've done? I thought to myself. *Is that what this is?*

I looked around to the crowds of people. I watched them shuffle as they looked down at their phones. I saw others gathering for photos, adjusting their hair. I heard cameras clicking. The garbage can was overflowing with Styrofoam containers and plastic bottles. I watched a small child as they dropped a toy over the edge of the boardwalk. Their parents didn't notice. Where were their parents?

"Can I go back to the car?" asked a teenager, in a petulant whine. "I want to watch a movie."

A lot of people say that the complexity of our languages combined with our unique communication abilities is what makes a human a human. I tend to agree that we're rather extraordinary when it comes to this, but I think we're more extraordinary at something else—I think human beings are masterful when it comes to forgetting. Given our undeniable advantages when it comes to mental capacity, the regularity with which we forget astounds me. Nature does not do this. It has no choice but to remember—to know, to be, and to express the fullness of its self.

What makes us uniquely human is that we can be something that we're not. We can unlearn our essence. We can forget. We can ebb away from ourselves, forever if we choose to.

Yes, we have lost track of ourselves. Yes, we think we're bigger than her. Yes, we are forgetting who and what we are.

My insides shake at the idea of this. At the thought that this isn't just about my mother and me, but all of us. That we might be participating in the greatest mass forgetting in history, a collective emptying of memory banks, a hollowing of our essence so large and so consuming that it threatens to break us all, not just those who have Alzheimer's, not just their families with them.

We've been relying on our brains for far too long. And now, it seems they are collapsing under the weight of it all. No longer able to keep what we demanded they promise—which was to make the world certain, and safe, and known.

I wonder what it will take for us to return to ourselves? To rush back to shore, our hands full of droplets of water, the bits of essence we'd flicked from our fingertips? I wonder if we will make ourselves whole again—if we will step back into not our personhood or our staunch individuality, but our kinship and connection, our very human nature.

I squeezed my mother's hand and looked out over the springs.

"It looks like the ground was split open," she said. "I wonder if someone will come and sew it back up."

"Maybe you can," I said. "You used to sew all the time."

"I did?" she asked, searching her brain for evidence of needles and thread, for the faint hum of a sewing machine. "I don't remember doing that."

"You made the curtains in the den," I offered as a reminder. "And a lot of our clothes. Especially when Christina and Charlie were little."

She paused. Something was making its way to the surface. Something was being remembered.

"And the Halloween costumes," she added.

"Yes," I confirmed. "The Halloween costumes. Like the stoplight. I think all four of us wore the stoplight."

I'm not sure how long it will take us to shift our gaze away from the things we believe to be ours—the people and places—so as to look toward the expanse of beauty waiting just around the corner. It seems there is a wildly peaceful place waiting for us on those planes, a place infused with a kind of sprawling vulnerability, that kind that only settles in after having experienced complete and utter exposure of who and what we really are. It seems there is belonging for us there. Remembrance of our deepest connections.

And perhaps my friend Maia had been correct in her equation. Perhaps children who survive an era of forgetting will be seen to have the medicine of remembrance.

"I hope so," I heard from a voice whispering up my skin.

This was the beginning of understanding something I knew I would never understand. It was the doorway into the feminine—a grotto of faith, a place where deep-seated knowing and exuberant curiosity live together like mother and daughter.

This was how I was returned to my mother—an arrival at the threshold of my thousand miles of wilderness, my refusal to be tamed.

20

With Earth as My Witness

Our flight was set to leave very early the next morning, so I wanted us fed, packed, and in bed earlier than normal. I looked at the clock on the dashboard of the car. It was just after four o'clock, and we were only a few minutes from downtown Bozeman. Perfect timing for an early dinner.

We both ordered salads and they were huge—each one seemed big enough for a family of four to share. I ate until I was well over full—about half the salad—and then watched as my mom cleaned her plate.

"You were hungry!" I said, as she used her fork to scrape her bowl clean.

She looked at me and smiled, placing her fork back down on the table.

"Yummy in my tummy," she said.

I paid the bill, and we hopped back into the car, our early-to-bed plans on track. It was just after five.

"Where next?" asked my mom.

"To the hotel," I said. "We're going to stay at a hotel to-night before we catch a flight home in the morning. It's right close to the airport."

She buckled her seat belt.

"Home?" she asked. "We're all done? We go home now?"

"Yep. We go home tomorrow."

"Oh," she said flatly. "No more tenting?"

"No more tenting," I replied.

We remained silent for the rest of the drive.

When we got to the hotel, we loaded up a luggage trolly with all of our gear and brought everything up to our room. My mom placed her purse on the coffee table, helped unload the trolly, and then glanced at her watch.

"Six o'clock," she announced. "I guess it's time for dinner."

I started to laugh. I was still stuffed from what we had inhaled just an hour or so earlier.

"Mom," I said. "We already had dinner."

"We did?" she asked. "When? It's only six."

I paused.

"Mom?" I asked slowly.

"Uh-huh."

"Are you hungry? Are you hungry for dinner?"

She paused too. I could see her thinking. Processing. The right side of her mouth moved upward ever so slightly.

"Well. I'm not sure," she said. "When was the last time we ate?"

"That part doesn't matter, Mom. I just want to know if you're hungry. Do you feel hungry?"

She went to look at her watch again, and I reached out and took her hand. I looked her in the eye.

"Are you hungry?" I asked, a little more firmly.

"I don't know. I think so," she said.

I didn't expect my mother to remember the restaurant we had been to. Nor did I expect her to be able to recall what we had eaten or if she had actually eaten. I was used to that— the loss of her cognitive memory, her not remembering the events of the day. But this was new. This marked an entrance into a whole new landscape—the loss of sensations, the loss of cues that moved through her body.

Is this how it works? I thought to myself. *Is this the progression?*

It was. My mother's brain would continue to lose things—a never-ending sieve that was working to filter her all the way out of herself. And it began recruiting her body for help. The pair would work in tandem for the next handful of years, sifting, sifting, sifting—losing every bit of the language I was just now learning.

I sat down on the edge of the bed in the hotel room and I cried. I felt like I had just watched Alzheimer's place a piece of cheesecloth over top of my mother's own heart, preparation for a long, slow strain until everything was gone but her skin.

"Why are you crying?" she asked.

"Because I love you, Mom," I said. "I'm crying because I love you."

"Well, that doesn't seem like a good thing to cry about," she said, her voice laced with confusion.

I laughed.

"Oh," she said, laughing along with me, teasing. "My little baby, crying because she loves me."

It was the first time on this trip that she referred to me as one of her kids—knew me, and named me as her daughter, her youngest, her baby.

Through the laughter I cried even harder. She walked over and tentatively sat down beside me, placing one of her hands on my knee.

"Don't be sad," she said, as she peered at me, attempting to catch my eye.

I looked up and saw worry marking her face—sweet, yet sorrowful eyes, a slight furrow in her brow, her mouth held in the shape of a silent coo.

It was one of the last times I remember being loved by my mother. The last time I saw that look sweep across her face. Her love always came through thickest when woven together with worry. I remember, for a split second, wondering who would take over, thinking about who would fill the void of loving me, worrying about me, seeing me through to some sort of end.

An answer came by way of my words.

"It's okay, Mom," I told her. "It's okay to be sad. It's okay to be sad," I repeated softly, not sure if I was telling her or reminding myself.

I would take over. I would love me. I would see myself through to some sort of end. This felt true to me, but also, as though something was missing.

My mother nodded gently and then looked down at her watch.

"Oooh," she said. "It's just after six. What are we doing for dinner?"

I took a deep breath in, explained that we had already eaten, and asked if, instead, she wanted to help me pack. We spent the next hour or so sorting out our various bags and getting rid of the things we couldn't take on our flight. We were zipped up and in bed by eight o'clock.

My mom fell asleep right away, but I stayed up. I stared at the ceiling for an hour or so, wishing it was the mesh and nylon rain fly of our tent, wishing the whirring noise of the hotel air conditioner was aspen leaves rustling in the breeze. I wasn't ready to leave the wilderness behind. The wilderness outside of myself and the wilderness inside of myself, the vast expanse I was standing on the cusp of, just now beginning to glimpse.

My mother lived in the wilderness, and for my whole life she had been calling me like a whispering robin to join her there.

I was terrified of this place, to both go there and be left alone there. It was the reason I built walls and busied myself. It was the reason I filled the world around me, and inside of me, with a cacophony of noise. It was the reason I wanted so badly for my mother to talk and talk some more—so I would not feel so alone in this stunning but savage place, in this, a waking human life.

I don't think I'm the only one who fears this. I think most of us are scared of being awake in the wilderness; the idea that we might run into some howling beast on the trails sends shivers up our spines. But we have it all wrong, for the most terrifying part is the silence, the immensity of the unknown, the idea that we might find something wholly unfamiliar in the shadows. Because only in that kind of stillness can we see the truth, can we discover that we are the howling beasts on the trails, and that nature is just a mirror, a reflection of everything deeply silent and yet wailing within us.

As I lay there that night the wilderness didn't seem that scary anymore. And I so badly wanted to go back, to go in. I felt I'd barely begun to see what was there, never mind come to know and understand it. And I recognized that my mother had prepared me for this place, that she had given me everything I needed to thrive within it, to understand that the velvety shadows around me were simply a reflection. And all I had to do was close my eyes and feel my way through. All I had to do was recognize myself in the darkness.

We boarded an early flight the next morning from Bozeman direct to Vancouver. My mother drank a cranberry juice and colored for the first handful of hours or so, while I read a book in the seat beside her.

About halfway through the flight she turned to look at me.

"Hi," she said, cheerily.

"Hi," I said back.

"You were a good mommy," she added.

I stared at her, wondering where this was going.

"You took good care of me," she said. "I'm your baby-mommy now."

I didn't know what to say. I didn't want to be anyone's mommy. I didn't want to be my mother's mommy.

I grabbed her hand, squeezed it gently, and smiled. As I looked at her, a memory from a few years prior edged itself into my mind—my mother and I, sitting with my grandmother at her dining room table.

It was sometime in the year or so before my mom and all of her sisters moved my grandmother into a care home. Her dementia had progressed far enough that she needed help with things like shopping, and laundry, the writing and sending of birthday cards. My mom and my aunts took turns visiting, helping my grandmother with various things, and I happened to be in town on one of the days my mother was set to go see her. It was "check-writing" day. The process was slow and tedious, and my mother was restless, a sure sign of her frustration.

My grandmother asked who the check should be written out to multiple times. My mother repeated the information over and over again. My grandmother would get distracted, causing her to have to ask again. I remember watching my mother as she fought back the urge to pull the checkbook away from her mother and just write the damn things herself.

Partway through the process, my grandmother turned to me—her green eyes were soft like liquid jade.

"She takes good care of me," she said, before turning to my mother.

"You take care of me, don't you?" she asked.

My mom's shoulders fell. She didn't want to be her mother's mommy. She took a deep breath.

"Yes, Mom," she said. "I take good care of you."

They smiled at one another. I saw my grandmother's hand resting on top of her right pant leg, her fingers moving over top of the material in small circles.

"Now," said my grandmother. "Who is this to again?"

As I looked at my mom on the plane, I noticed her other hand, the one I wasn't holding. It was resting on her tray table, on the cocktail napkin the flight attendant had given to her. My mother's fingers were moving over the top of the napkin in small circles.

Have we been drawing a map to get back to one another? I wondered. *To get back to ourselves?*

No beginning. No end. Everyone and everything encompassed.

"You are found here," it would read. "In the center of it all. In the center of yourself."

My dad was waiting for us in the passenger pickup zone of the airport. Luggage was loaded into the back of the car, and there were quick hugs and kisses before we climbed in and drove home. Once there, we ate a quick lunch and settled into the sand-colored couches in my parents' living room, late afternoon sun streaming through the windows.

"So . . ." said my dad with excitement, as he turned to me and then to my mom, "what were the highlights?"

I looked at my mom. Her face was completely blank. I watched as the question hit her, and perhaps it was less the question and more the fact that she was supposed to have an answer for it. She scanned her brain. Nothing. She smiled an awkward smile.

"It was wonderful," she said, as she gently placed each of her hands on the tops of her thighs. "All of it was wonderful."

And with that it was gone. Our whole trip, erased in entirety. It was as if a deposit had never been made. As if pages from a journal had suddenly gone missing.

All in all, my mom and I had been on the road for eleven days. We drove 1,957 miles through three states and three glorious national parks. We saw seven bears, eleven if you include the ones I dreamt about. We slept in five different campsites, we went through two bottles of Baileys, and I learned, slowly and fitfully, the definition of surrender, or at least the first few steps. I had walked, holding my mother's hand as she led the way into the stony silence of the wilderness, only to realize that there is more aliveness there than anywhere I had ever been.

And there was my mother, unable to recall a single second of it.

And there I was, sitting on the couch in the home I grew up in, flooded with memories, with clues about how to find myself, and with questions about who would hold my hand in the cavernous darkness.

It was a trip my mother will never remember and a journey I'll never forget.

What happens now? I wondered to myself. *What on earth happens now?*

I had one more night at my parents' house before my flight back to California, and that question circled like a hawk in my brain. I felt as though the trip with my mother had served as some sort of introductory lesson—like I now knew the first two or three silent words in the lexicon of the Universe, but I had no idea what came next, or, as my mother continued to fade, who would take over as my teacher.

As I washed my face that night, I felt those hawks soaring, yet again, on the thermals inside of me. After I rinsed and dried my face, I held the towel in my wet hands and I looked into the mirror, wondering, hoping perhaps, that the face looking back at me would have all the answers. I leaned in and stared. I still couldn't see much more than a trace of my mother. So I leaned in further, yearning for something, some additional clue that she had tucked into the fabric of me. But I didn't see it.

My shoulders slumped forward in disappointment and I got back to drying my hands. As I hung the towel up, I could have sworn I heard a voice:

Pinch them, it said. *Pinch the tops of your hands.*

I laughed.

Sure. What the heck, I thought to myself, as I grabbed a bit of skin on the top of my left hand.

I pulled gently and let it go, watching it move back down at a medium pace. And as I watched I noticed something else—my hands, my nails, the small wrinkles that gently arced across my knuckles. I turned my hands over and looked at the soft pads of my fingertips, and the lines that ran side to side, up and down, diagonally across on my palms.

It was all there. Everything I had been looking for. Fingerprints were mountain ranges, small, whirling topographical maps. The deep lines on my palms were canyons and gorges, and braided riverbeds. Blue veins that ran faintly under the surface of the tops of my hands were underground channels, narrow aquifers where groundwater was able to flow. I touched the inside of my forearm, just underneath my wrist—the skin was soft, almost silky, like finely tilled silt.

I may not look like my mother, I thought to myself. *But I do look like Mother Nature.*

And with that, my teacher appeared. Ocean tides and shooting stars. Old-growth forests and the sound of wind moving through grassland. Mountaintops and river bottoms. Storms that rage across plains. Lightning bolts that split the sea. It all made sense—for the only mother bigger than my own is Mother Nature.

In that moment, I knew I had to find my way back—not to the trip I'd just been on but to nature as a whole, to a life lived with her, to a place where my external world matched up with what I now knew existed inside of me. Where my life becomes not a reaction to mother but a co-creation with her. I needed to walk with earth as my witness, toward a place where the lines between myself and the divine blended and blurred, a place of connection and at-one-ment, where I could sit, nestled in the majesty of my lineage.

I looked back at myself in the mirror. I felt all of me nod in confirmation.

The journey with my mother was both complete and just beginning, which is, if you pay close enough attention, the way time has always unfolded.

Later that afternoon, my dad drove me to the airport so I could catch a flight back to Southern California. It was just the two of us in the car.

Just prior to the trip, my mother had seen a doctor to run a few tests, various things being measured so as to provide insight about her disease progression. I was curious to know if the results had come in while we were away, and if so, what they said. Not long into the drive to the airport, I asked.

"It's not great," said my dad in response, keeping his eyes on the road. "But I'm hoping she can still get into that trial."

"I thought she had to score below a certain number for that," I said. "Isn't she already well above that?"

He glanced at me before looking back to the road. I saw fleeting desperation in his eyes.

"Steph," he said sadly. "I just don't know what to do. I . . ." He paused and adjusted his grip on the steering wheel. "I guess I'm just hoping for a miracle here."

As Anne Lamott wrote: "It's a little late for beggy prayers. It's time for trust and surrender."

"Dad," I said. "I mean, I'm not going to tell you *not* to ask for a miracle, but don't you see?"

"See what?" he asked.

"We've already lived one," I said. "We've lived a thousand of them."

He grabbed my hand and gave it two quick squeezes—the rhythm of a singular heartbeat. We spent the rest of the drive in silence. Not a word from the two most talkative people in the bloodline. Because there is nothing more wild than silence. My mother, she taught me that lesson.

My mother is a miracle. She is a thousand of them. She runs like a river, coursing through all of our veins.

Of all the wisdom I've garnered in my life, this is the singular piece I hope to retain: I am nothing without her and everything with her.

Epilogue

Standing on the Shore

In the five and a half years since the trip with my mother, I have dreamt of bears every June. That month seems to serve as some sort of marker—my mother and the sky above her conspiring, sending signals, an interstellar Morse code to my subconscious. June of 2020 was no different.

The dream came early in the month, around the sixth or the seventh. In it, I came across a large bear. It was sprawled across a section of pavement just outside the entrance to a hospital.

The bear began to pant and I noticed its tongue and its gums—pale pink, almost white. It was exhausted. It was dehydrated. It was alive, but barely.

I walked closer to it, and, without raising its head, the bear looked up at me. Its eyes were pleading. It could not walk, or crawl, or pull itself one step further, but it was clear to me that the bear was attempting to make it inside the hospital. It couldn't say it out loud, but the bear needed care. I looked around for help, and suddenly a large man dressed in blue appeared. Together, we carried the bear through the doors. Once inside, the bear was placed on a gurney and whisked away. Its condition was critical. I stayed back to check the bear in, to provide the details I knew.

After asking me its name (unknown), its age (unknown), its blood type (also unknown), the woman behind the desk reached over the counter, took my hands, and said, "Don't worry. Your mother will be just fine. We've got her now. We've got her."

One month later, almost to the day, my mother was moved into a full-time care facility in Vancouver, Canada. I could feel her relief from 150 miles away, where I live now, tucked into a grove of large cedars. I could feel my mother's deliverance, her wild and joyful freedom. Wordlessly, silently, it moved through the ground, through the roots, the mycorrhiza of all the trees that are rooted into the soil between my mother and me, the bloodred veins that connect us.

Because of coronavirus-based border closures and quarantine rules, as well as the sound health and safety precautions put in place by my mother's care facility, I have not seen her for well over a year. And I'm not sure, but it may be much longer.

A part of me is deeply saddened by this. But another part, the part that speaks the language of silence, the part that knows how to pick up words on the wind, is at peace. Because I know that my mother is everywhere.

She is coiled up inside my DNA. She is in the bedrock of the earth. I find her in every layer of soil and silt around me and underneath me. She is inside every crevice of every rock I see; she is trickling through every stream. My mother is groundwater, searching for paths, moving swiftly now out to the ocean, and I am the landscape being carved in her wake. I will stand on the shore and watch her cut sand. Ever after, my eyes will be trained on the water.

My mother is everywhere, as is her mother. I find the pair of them in the jagged peaks of the mountains around me, in the clouds that form above me. They are the faces carved into a large stone near my house—an ancient altar with a silent story. I am the person who visits, who sits and prays at their feet. I can hear their laughter inside the chittering sound of the eagles who live by the beach. I can see the women of my lineage in the eyes of the family of deer before they bounce shyly away with a wee fawn in tow. They're everywhere, which makes me think I might be too.

A lot of people might say it took me a long time to come to this—the idea that divinity lives both inside of us and all around us. But to see it that way would be both narrow-sighted and narrow-minded. Because in actual fact, it has taken millennia. It takes time to rise. It takes eons and earthquakes. It takes glaciated ice scraping down your back, thousands of years of stony pressure. It takes water dripping, one droplet a day for a million days, and then a million more. It takes the heat of a culture that wants to burn you down. It takes the lingering heat of a culture that has.

You see, a woman doesn't rise on her own. She does it through lineage. She does it by placing her life on top of her mother's, and so on and so forth for thousands of years. I am but a tiny hill, but when you add me to my mother, and to her mother before her, we begin to form a mountain. When you add all of us together, we are Everest, or as the Nepali say, "Goddess of the Sky."

I am the evolution of my mother. She is the backbone I am growing into. The two of us, along with hundreds who came before us, form a collective, and this . . . this has been our hundred thousand–year rise, our merging into a singular chain of starlight that pours down from the sky.

Never have I felt like more of myself. Never have I felt more whole, more powerful, more like her, more like me, more like some intoxicating blend of the both of us, and the ones who came before. All of us now, moving in the same direction at once, dancing together on the shore after decades at sea.

Some things may be forgotten. But in the process, we shall be remembered.

Acknowledgments

Every book comes with a mycorrhizal network, an underground web that provides nourishment pertinent to the book's creation. I am indebted to the below list of people, my underground web, without whom this book would not have broken the ground of me, nor I the ground of it.

To Sarah J. Murphy, few people in my life have the ability to see me as I am in any particular moment as well as where I am capable of going. You are one of them. You have illuminated so much in my life. May the cycle of the full moon continue to show us the way.

To Bryn Clark, few people in my life have the ability to see the future me and ask me to be her now. You are one of them. You have planted many seeds within me as well as in my work. May the cycle of the new moon continue to show us the way.

To the entire team at Flatiron, being a sapling in the forest you've so carefully grown is both humbling and inspiring. To be planted with you fills me with gratitude and a sense of possibility.

To my agent, Laura Yorke, thank you for believing I am

capable of going to the place where the stars are aligned and the cosmos are created. Your support has meant the world.

Kristina Oldani, you once wrote to me about how chaos from up close disappears into a larger scene of becoming when we allow space and time to swell. Thank you for bearing witness and for encouraging me to fold that very notion into every blank space I encounter, on the page or otherwise.

To Maia Toll, who tugged on *the* most important thread at *the* most important time—this book would not be what it is without you. Your support at the finish line was invaluable. Your support beyond the finish line is something I cherish.

To Sarah Selecky, whose camaraderie and wisdom I have treasured. To all of the women in all of my writing groups, past and present. To Bretty Rawson and Joyce Chen, for continuing to create and hold an unnamable space. Thank you.

To my Owl Rebels—Kaki, Kylie, Madison, Erin, and Geraldine—that year you all learned to walk in the dark fed this book in immeasurable ways. Deepest bow.

Shannah Crane Dimmick, you hold so much steady as I move here and there and everywhere. I do better work, and I am a much better person, with you in my life. Gold star for you!

To Janet Bertolus, I don't have words. Just the smell of gardenia and the taste of black licorice, the sound of a knee being slapped in the distance. You are my Yaltha. You have taught me so much about love and the art of trespassing.

To my family (and to all of the families impacted by Alzheimer's and dementia), I'm so sorry we're here, but I'm glad we're all here together. With one another, this is excruciating.

Without one another, it's impossible. Thank you for the all the ways in which you've shown up, shared your stories and cared for mine.

To Chris, my beloved, you have helped me build a place in which I can be everything, where every piece of me is allowed to exist. I am whole because of you, not because you're my better half, but because you've spent over a decade encouraging me to find all of myself. And this book, we both know it had to be written from all of myself.

To my father, the most valuable lessons you have given me (and there have been many) are the ones about silver linings. This book would not exist, and she would not have become what she became, if you had not taught me how to search for, build and rebuild life around those kinds of threads. I love you.

Last, to my mother . . . your greatest gift to the world was the way in which you mothered. I have come to believe that this book is your way of continuing that work—mothering anyone who reads but a word of it. Your life as a cedar was a spectacular thing to both behold and be part of. But your life now, as a great and grand nursing log, mothering the whole of the ancient forest, is nothing short of miraculous. I am so proud to be one of your daughters.

About the Author

Steph Jagger is a sought-after mentor and coach whose offerings guide people toward a deeper understanding of themselves and their stories. Her work, including speaking and facilitating, lies at the intersection of loss, the nature of deep remembrance, and the personal journey of re-creation. Steph lives and works on Bainbridge Island, Washington. Her first book, *Unbound*, was published in 2017.